Z-FAST:

A Simple, Proven Intermittent Fasting Method

By
John Zehren

Second printing July 2018

Edited by Marlayna Glynn and Stacy Shawn

Interior design by Dave Scott

Cover design by Diren Yardimli

Contact the author Johnny Z: www.zfast.us

Dedicated to my parents Roger & Peggy Zehren

CONTENTS

Z–FAST: A Simple, Proven Intermittent Fasting Method

INTRODUCTION

Hey, I'm John Zehren, creator of Z-FAST.

I'm just a regular guy with a wife and kids, a busy career, and a fun social life.

In the eight years since I PERMANENTLY lost the extra weight I'd picked up since college, I became informally known as, "Johnny Z, that fasting guy."

How did this happen?

Well, first I got "fat."

I didn't much like it, and my wife didn't care for it either.

I tried all that diet stuff, and it just didn't work for me, just like it doesn't work for most folks.

I couldn't be bothered with equipment, portioning, special diets, extended targeted workouts, specialized meals, or the high costs of name-brand diet food.

I had NO time to exercise.

I had NO time to diet.

I only had time NOT to EAT.

So, I decided to do my own thing, and follow a method of intermittent fasting a few times per month, cycling between periods of eating and fasting.

It wasn't about what to eat, but rather when NOT to eat.

It sounds crazy, but it worked: I lost the weight and kept it off.

FOR EIGHT YEARS.

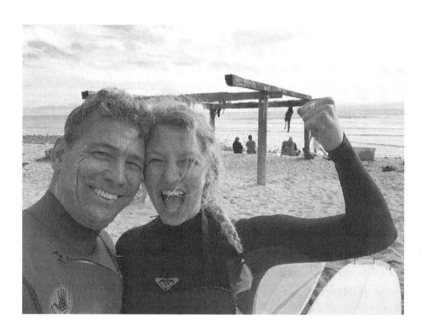

A HEALTHY, HAPPY, FASTER who is full of energy again.
I'm surfing and keeping up with my 22-year-old daughter.

That's unusual.

Not because I am unusual (well, it depends who you ask), but that I was able to keep the weight off.

See, not only do most dieters regain the original weight they lose, but the National Institute of Health reports that one-third to two-thirds of dieters regain more weight than was dropped on their diets![1]

It's a vicious cycle that happens to be pretty tough on the poor old body. When you lose weight and gain it back, it's worse for the body than if you had done nothing at all.

And I know you know what I'm talking about.

I don't possess a great deal of discipline when it comes to continuously portioning my food on a daily basis for life (like all the other diet fads require you to do).

I can't have one handful of chips when I want three, or ease off on some killer 7-layer dip because it's high in fat. I can't drink one beer when I'd prefer two. I can't have a glass of orange juice because I'll overstep my "caloric intake."

And I can never say no to that birthday cake!

It doesn't work for me to suffer, and I know it doesn't work for you either. I need food and wine in my life, and I'd rather shut it down once or twice a month and eat regularly the rest of the time.

You know, that whole "eat, drink, and be merry" thing.

That's why I created the Z-FAST.

---

[1] "Prevalence of Obesity Among Adults and Youth: United States, 2011–2014." Centers for Disease Control and Prevention, Centers for Disease Control and Prevention, 28 Oct. 2015, www.cdc.gov/nchs/data/databriefs/db219.html

I had to slam the door on calories, turn on weight loss, and kick my fat-burning machine into high gear!

Instead of "dieting," I learned I could fast to achieve a lifetime of health benefits while reaching a weight I am proud to maintain.

Z-FAST is the easiest approach yet because you only need two pieces of equipment: a calendar and a scale.

Don't worry; I'll provide easy-to-follow instructions, as well as the new scientific proof of the merits of intermittent fasting. Buckle up (and I do mean tighten your belt buckle!) because Z-FASTING will allow you to unleash the energy you need (and already have stored right in your body) ... your fat!

There are three simple fasting methods I'll explain which you can follow to reach and maintain your optimum weight for a healthier and happier life. Here's a brief overview, so you'll know what to expect by using a combination of these three methods.

(I will explain the Z-FAST method in greater detail in Chapter Eleven.)

INTRODUCING THE Z-FAST METHODS

THE SYSTEMATIC FAST is used to lose a significant amount of weight such as 10–50 pounds, and to reach your lifetime commitment weight (more on that later.)

You can continue your regular weekend eating and drinking on your off days while holding true to your fast days and STILL drop the pounds.

THE SCHEDULED FAST is used for those seeking to maintain weight after the Systematic Fast. This approach follows a calendared schedule with one full fast day per month, and three half fasts per month (breakfast and lunch skipped).

THE INTERVENTION FAST is used for those determined never to gain pounds again. This "when needed fast" is critical to keep the lifetime commitment weight and stay under your promised weight.

That's all there is to it.

Prepare yourself for immediate results!

Say no to food and yes to benefits.

With Z-FAST, there is no portioning, no massive exercise programs, no special foods or menus, no added time and energy to DO SOMETHING. This is about doing LESS. It's much easier than any other "diet," and you have everything you need to get started tomorrow.

No prepping, no planning, no shopping.

One of the best parts of Z-FAST is that you don't have to change your life on weekends or on the days when you're not fasting.

No schlepping around plastic tubs of "your food" to parties.

Those dried-out, stringy celery stalks on the chicken wing platter at the company banquet won't be your lunch.

No sweating at that summer barbecue and chewing ice while you wish you could drink a cold one with your pals.

That slice of birthday cake at celebrations is all yours.

Happy hour with the work colleagues has your name on it!

For the most part, you can continue the same eating regimen you now follow. Reducing more calories helps, but is not necessary.

Of course, you don't want to go crazy, and binge eat when you're not fasting. You should, of course, exert some reasonableness on your non-fasting days.

This could mean a smaller piece of cake, fewer handfuls of chips, or drinking less alcohol to get even more of a benefit.

But you can still enjoy these goodies and don't need to eliminate them entirely from your life. And if you do "blow it" … there's THE INTERVENTION Z-FAST to your rescue! (That's exactly what it's for.)

Aside from being an effective way to lose weight, the Z-FAST comes with some super-power health benefits beyond weight loss that I'll discuss in detail including an improved fat burning process, metabolism increases, lowered risk for heart disease, improved ability to fight and possibly prevent cancer, heightened awareness and focus and increased longevity.[2]

[2] "Are There Any Proven Benefits to Fasting?" *Johns Hopkins Health Review,* www.johnshopkinshealthreview.com/issues/spring-summer-2016/articles/are-there-any-proven-benefits-to-fasting

3 Intermittent Fasting Methods: Z-FAST

01

Z-FAST Systematic: Major Weight Loss
- 1/2-day fast 1 time per week
- Full Fast 1 time per week
- Normal eating outside fast days

02

Scheduled Z-FAST: Maintain Your Weight
- Weekly 1/2-day fast
- 1 full-day fast once a month
- Spontaneous fasting

03

Z-FAST Intervention: Lifetime Weight Commitment
- Immediate fast when over your commitment weight
- Keep your promise
- Weigh yourself daily

Ho et al. (1988). "Fasting enhances growth hormone secretion and amplifies the complex rhythms of growth hormone secretion in man." *The Journal of Clinical Investigation*. 1988 Apr; 81(4); 968–975. DOI: 10.1172/JCI113450.
www.ncbi.nlm.nih.gov/pmc/articles/PMC329619

Hartman et al. (1992). "Augmented growth hormone (GH) secretory bursts frequency and amplitude mediate enhanced GH secretion during a two-day fast in normal man." *The Journal of Clinical Endocrinology and Metabolism*. 1992 Apr; 74(4); 757–765. DOI 10.1210/jcem.74.4.1548337.
www.ncbi.nlm.nih.gov/pubmed/1548337

Weight loss plus health benefits — what's not to like?

Exercise benefits are compounded.

You can also continue your regular exercise program (I'll explore this in Chapter Eight) and obtain the double benefit of exercising while fasting because your body releases extra healthy hormones.

Human growth hormones (HGH) increase an astounding 2,000% in men and 1,300% in women when fasting![3]

You're going to read a lot about HGH because this is critical for building a healthy body, especially in promoting muscle growth, libido in women, tissue repair, and muscle tone.

If you decide not to exercise, you'll still experience the weight loss and fat burn because when you reduce caloric intake while fasting, you lose stored fat and pounds. It's inevitable!

In contrast to old-school thinking, fasting has been scientifically shown to increase metabolism[4] while burning fat stores. Where else would your body get energy if there is no blood sugar from the continuous feeding of calories other than from stored fat? That's one of the secrets of fasting: FAT BURN!

---

[3] "Fasting and growth hormone." Diet Doctor, 15 Dec. 2017, www.dietdoctor.com/fasting-and-growth-hormone

[4] "10 Evidence-Based Health Benefits of Intermittent Fasting." Healthline, Healthline Media, www.healthline.com/nutrition/10-health-benefits-of-intermittent-fasting

Intermittent Fast Advantages

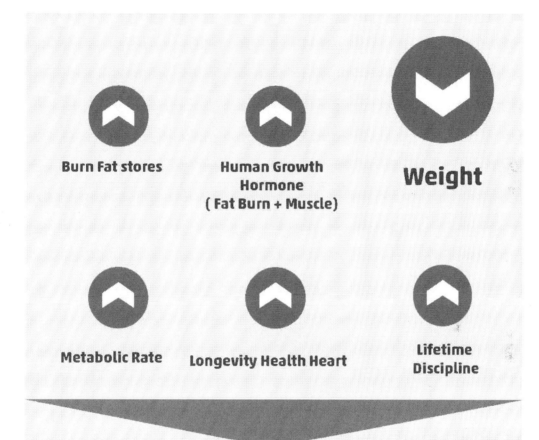

Burn Fat stores

Human Growth Hormone
(Fat Burn + Muscle)

Weight

Metabolic Rate

Longevity Health Heart

Lifetime Discipline

Human Growth Hormone:

1) 2,000% increase in a study from the "American College of Cardiology" on Fasting
2) Promotes muscle growth, libido, tissue repair, boosts fat loss and increases metabolism

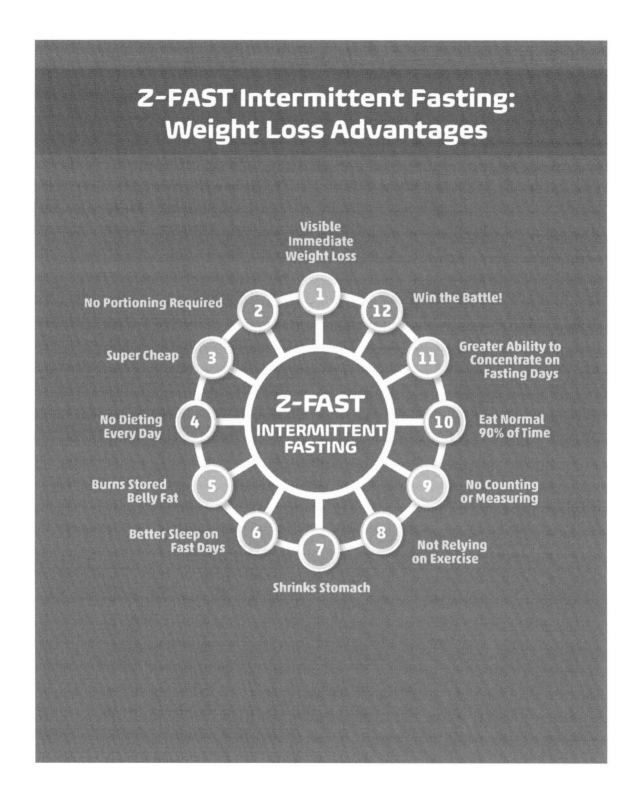

Slam the door on calories and activate your fat-burning machine!

Your body will activate the process to go after the fat stores and retrieve it and use it for energy as it is the next available energy source.

(That's why fat stores are there, waiting for when the body needs them).

Z-FAST is the ultimate fat-burning system.

When you follow the method I lay out in the subsequent chapters and commit to the intermittent fasting lifestyle, you will not only burn off that unwanted weight, but you'll maintain your optimal weight while reaping documented health benefits as well.

I invite you to give it a shot!

The advantages are numerous! Fasting is the easiest path to health and weight loss for life!

CHAPTER ONE

My Slow and Unstoppable Weight Gain

"I fast for greater physical and mental efficiency."

— Plato

I'm no Plato.

As I said, I'm just a regular guy.

By that I mean I live in a crazy, busy world whizzing around me at a ridiculous rate. I balance three kids, a wife, a mortgage, a high-pressure job managing a lot of people, and a traffic-packed commute to and from the office in Southern California.

(And did I mention the three daughters?)

Plus, I travel a lot which means I don't have a standard schedule.

And when I am at home, I need to keep up with the house, attend my daughters' games and performances, enjoy the neighborhood barbecues, struggle through that dang traffic, and interact on social media and the internet which demand that I answer hundreds of text messages and emails EVERY DAY.

This goes on 24 hours a day, seven days a week. You can probably relate.

As I gained weight, I soon found I was too busy to diet, count calories, measure portions, buy particular products or equipment, or schedule time with a personal trainer.

I only wanted to enjoy my life, my family, and my work!

There was no time in the day for me to dedicate to my health if that required that I eliminate something else I needed to do. I found it hard to cut out a great party, one of the kids' events, or a chance to improve at the office.

I needed to be sharp enough to deliver at work and show up for my family and my community, and that made it hard to find any extra time to exercise for potential health gains.

Initially, as the weight started creeping on, I tried to diet and exercise. I really did.

But I just couldn't seem to find a way to cut things out of my life that made me happy to create time for scheduled exercise or shopping for the latest diet craze.

All of these challenges got me into a tight place that I found unsettling.

You can see my life weight from age 18-54 illustrated in the chart that follows. I started at 167 pounds, peaked at 205 pounds, and after a Z-FAST intervention, went down to 185 pounds, a weight I've maintained for eight years now.

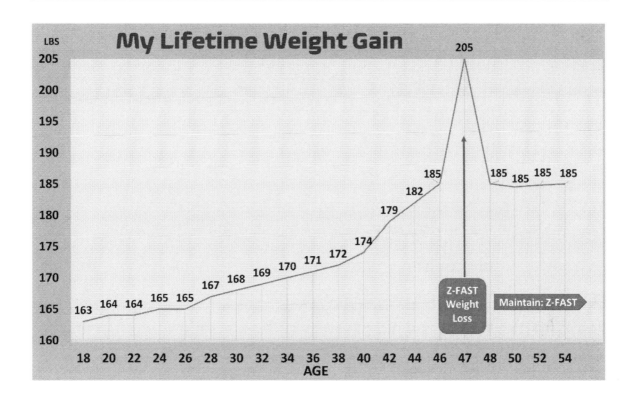

Peaking at 205 lbs, I initiated the Systematic Z-FAST weight loss method and lost 20+ lbs. Using the methods in this book, I've kept it off for eight years.

In high school, I set a pole vaulting record at my 164-pound weight!

(Yeah, I know. Glory days.)

When I turned 40, it was like the "weight gain" switch had been flipped in my body, and my normal lifestyle began to work against me.

I became sedentary with my desk job.

(Sadly, no opportunities for pole vaulting there! Only pencil-pushing.)

The burger and chips I wolfed down at a friend's barbecue meant I would be tipping the scales the very next day.

The drink or two I imbibed at a client dinner meant a bigger tire around my belly.

A family birthday party meant my pants would be tighter the next morning.

My metabolism slowed down as my weight gain sped up.

It became harder to lose weight, and, alarmingly easier to put it on.

Some of you know *INSIDIOUS* as a series of horror flicks, but INSIDIOUS to me is the horror story of how weight crept up on me.

Now that was scary!

At first, it was an additional pound every four months, which didn't seem like a big deal. What's wrong with a measly three pounds a year?

Then it increased to two pounds in the next six months.

Add another three pounds every three or four months.

Over the course of two or three years, I had "suddenly" picked up more than 20 pounds.

BAM! I was overweight and unhappy.

In the midst of feeling bad about myself, I was also undergoing a cross-country job relocation and promotion, while doing my best to focus 100% on my family and day-to-day work.

As my weight gain continued, for the next two years I tried many diet strategies to lose the pounds, including but not limited to:

- The Atkins diet (a few times)
- The "Zone" diet
- The "five-small-meals-a-day "diet
- The "no-bread" diet
- The "Hydroxycut" diet (the bottles are still in my drawer)
- The "skipping-dessert" diet
- The "half-portioning" diet
- The "skipping-the-heavy-sauces-and-creams" diet
- The "paleo" diet
- The "carb-counting" diet
- The "no-caloric-drinks" diet

See the common denominator in the above list?

They are all "diets," and NONE of them worked for me!

I did my best to fight weight-gain in the midst of my busy life, but like most Americans, the pounds just kept accumulating.

That small, inconsequential gain added up until I was undeniably overweight.

I was aware of the slow upward movement of my weight. But despite everything I tried, I was just unable to do anything but watch my weight gain spiral up.

I would lose two pounds with some diet or other and then gain it right back the very next week.

I would lose three pounds but then add seven at the neighborhood Super Bowl party. (At least that's how it felt.)

You get the picture.

You've been there too!

Finally, I tipped the scales at 200, and I was infuriated.

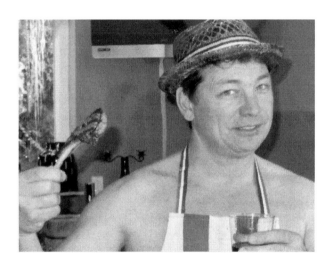

On a roll ... I slowly gained 20+ lbs. at 47 years old, my highest recorded weight of 205 lbs.

Ouch! I tried so hard not to get there.

I looked in the mirror and could not deny what was happening to me: love handles, tight pants, fat around my neck, and that "over forty" man belly.

NOOOO!

My days of looking good in a wetsuit were over!

But wait (weight!) there's more ...

As if 200 pounds wasn't bad enough, the scale crept up to 202, and then 205!

For the first time in my life, I was STUCK over 200 pounds and still gaining with no hope in sight.

It was as if worrying about weight gain was causing it.

So there I was in this loop of thought thinking about my weight at a time when I had a whole lot of other things to think about (like my daughters and my wife and my new job responsibilities).

I found myself worrying more and more about being overweight.

NO BUENO!

You could say I'm a pretty disciplined guy when I put my mind to something.

I know how to meet a goal.

Yet despite all my weight loss goal setting, I had nothing to show for it.

Well, that's not true. I had 25 pounds of weight gain to show for it.

Some people may not mind carrying an extra 25 pounds. They're happy, they feel good, and they don't mind buying new clothes. I respect that.

But not me. I didn't feel good or look good. I didn't feel healthy. Heck, I WASN'T healthy!

I should never have allowed myself to get to that point.

New suits and pants had to be ordered, as well as an exercise bike for the house.

I went on some sort of last-resort cabbage diet. And didn't lose a pound.

I stomped around the house, swearing at the scale and feeling grumpier than ever. Because of my crazy life, I had let myself go while riding the roller-coaster of ineffective diets.

I was in food hell. Everywhere I looked there was food: office parties, client dinners, big family meals, happy hours, birthday celebrations, and neighborhood parties.

Everything I had to do revolved around food, which meant I would gain even MORE weight!

It was terrible for me.

I became miserable, which didn't work for me or anyone around me.

I tried everything, and nothing was working.

I was so mad at myself. I just couldn't seem to change my whole lifestyle entirely and adhere to some new pattern.

And while kids are cute, they can be brutally honest. One of my young daughters asked me a profound question one day.

"Daddy, why are you still fat when you go on the scale every day?"

Out of the mouth of babes! That was it. That helped fuel my resolve to make a difference in my weight.

As innocent as the comment was, the beauty in it was that it was true, it was a fact, and it was helpful to motivate me.

As a husband, a father, and a manager at the office, I couldn't afford to be down and miserable, and I didn't want to be that overweight dad and husband.

I needed to stop the madness.

I was so done with that lifestyle.

I didn't have time to exercise (well, not enough to lose weight — more on that in Chapter Eight) and I didn't have time to manage and stick to a special diet.

But I did have time NOT to eat ... and that is where the weight loss magic finally happened.

Finally, I vowed, **"I am not going to eat one more morsel of food until I weigh less than 200 pounds."** And I lost five pounds ASAP.

And that, my friends, is how I stumbled upon THE FIRST FAST.

You're probably wondering how I finally managed to do it, and whether or not it was safe. **I had heard about fasting. And I had heard it was an effective tool for losing weight.**

So, I did my research.

I love science. I graduated cum laude with a degree in Biology from the University of St. Thomas in St. Paul, MN. For more than 35 years, I've worked in the medical and healthcare fields bringing new cures, and FDA-approved technologies to the market, specifically related to the heart and brain.

I'm currently the North American Vice President of Sales and on the management board for the neurovascular division of a major American healthcare company.

So the very first thing I did was hit the books. I had heard that humans had been fasting since Biblical times, but I had to know how long someone could go without food and what the side effects, drawbacks, and benefits might be. I had to make sure I could keep my promise to myself.

I learned that there is a multitude of well-documented cases of how long a person can go without food ranging from 21 days (Mahatma Gandhi) to a staggering medically supervised 382-day fast from the University Department of Medicine, Scotland. I certainly wasn't looking for anything that long. I was thinking 36 hours, so I knew I was good here.

All the extra food we eat becomes stored fat until needed, (that's the whole reason your body stores it!) The body first goes after that fat storage. Then the body moves on to muscle mass AFTER there is no fat left.

Remember this, because when you tell the naysayers you're fasting, they're going to say, "But fasting eats your muscles!"

NOT TRUE! (At least not until you've depleted all your fat stores.)

Water is a different story. You cannot survive much longer than three days without water.

It just so happened that my meltdown occurred on Fat Tuesday (some of you party animals might know this day as Mardi Gras), which immediately precedes Lent. Catholics celebrate Lent which symbolizes the biblical 40 days Jesus spent in the desert without eating.

Go ahead and laugh. I know. FAT TUESDAY.

(But it was my last Fat Tuesday!)

So, on the evening of Fat Tuesday, I committed to starting my first fast. The next day I skipped breakfast and headed out to work. Lunchtime rolled around, and I didn't eat then either. I had a headache, but I pushed through it. An afternoon cup of coffee took care of that.

By the time I came home my body was screaming, "I want food! Give me calories! Give me glucose!"

But I had committed to the fast and resolved to do something about my weight gain. I said no to dinner, leaving my wife confused as to why I didn't partake in the meal she had so lovingly prepared for me.

Evening rolled around, and I made it. And … it wasn't so bad.

Day One was on the books.

On Day Two of my fast, I skipped breakfast, lunch, and dinner again. Now I was at 48 hours with no food. I weighed myself, and I was almost at my goal of 200 pounds!

On Day Three I skipped breakfast and lunch. I finally, finally had dinner after this long fast (my first fast ever!)

I was under 200 pounds, and I felt GREAT!

I made it! I did it!

I felt empowered and was over the moon. I was amazed by the beneficial power of fasting. My thoughts were clear, and I didn't have the post-lunch nap time fatigue at the office.

I was on my game!

I realized I didn't need to eat all that much — certainly not as much as I had been eating.

And so I was inspired to keep going.

At 200 pounds, I began doing intermittent fasts where I skipped breakfast and lunch one day a week (half fast) and did one full fast day per week during the 40 days of Lent. (A full fast is no breakfast, lunch, or dinner by the way.)

Every Wednesday I fasted and chose another random day to skip breakfast and lunch.

At the end of Lent, I was down to 193 pounds after just six fasting days! And I lost real subcutaneous fat, not water weight.

So, I went another four weeks, fasting every Wednesday.

I noticed a huge benefit: when I did eat, I was eating far less than before.

In just 11 weeks of fasting each Wednesday, I reached my target weight of 185.0 — the same weight I enjoyed many years ago where I really felt good.

I made sure to get plenty of hydration and enjoy my usual dose of coffee.

If I felt like I was dragging later in the day, I would add another cup of coffee in the afternoon. (More on the benefits of coffee later.)

On this intermittent fasting schedule, I was able to hit 185.0 pounds after eleven weeks!

This was my lowest weight in years, and I loved it.

(And so did my wife!)

I was able to continue my regular lifestyle, which included exercising sporadically and eating regular meals. I only had to fast occasionally to maintain my desired weight.

During my fasting days, I made sure to drink a gallon of water and maybe drink an extra cup of coffee on an as-needed basis, but that was it.

Fasting took no time away from my busy schedule and my overwhelming number of obligations.

In fact, I couldn't believe how much time I saved because I wasn't continually prepping for a meal, worrying about a meal, planning for a meal, or going out for that "one-hour" lunch. Just eliminating the drive time was a bonus.

I found that I was much more productive when I fasted. I used the time it would have taken me to eat and put it back into my life.

This was a life-changing concept for me: losing weight and gaining time, with no fads, equipment, or special meals.

Hurrah for me!!

But wait, hold on ...

How would I maintain my weight loss? I'd been there before!

I knew I had to do something or I would fall victim to that subtle weight gain pattern again. I was faced with the all too common American dilemma: how would I keep the weight off?

Should I try the Zone diet again? Portion control?

Should I take one of those remaining $24 bottles of Hydroxycut that were still in my desk drawer?

Should I throw away all the ice cream, cookies, and fried chips in the pantry?

(I don't think my wife and daughters would have been too happy about that one!)

Should I go to a Halfway House for Fasters?

None of those options were genuinely viable, so I made what I called a LIFETIME COMMITMENT WEIGHT:

"I, Johnny Z, will never go above 185.0 pounds again."

That decimal is essential: in fact, it's the deal-breaker.

In the past, I would allow 185.6 or 185.9 to be "on track" for 185.0 pounds.

No problem.

I'd say, "Oh, a little water weight."

But then two weeks later I was up to 186.1.

The next day at 186.2, I would think it was more water weight, or I didn't go #2 that morning.

No problem.

Then I would be at 186.4.

That's barely a pound over, but then the weekend arrived, and I would be having a little dessert wine and goat cheese, a handful of chips, some salsa, a few cold ones and before I knew it, oops ... I was at 186.7 and had blown my whole systematic fasting success and goal of 185.0 that I'd worked so hard to reach.

Just like that, I was over my goal weight of 185.0. (Remember the importance of that decimal!)

And so the American insidious weight gain cycle would continue ...

Again.

Again?

Not on my watch!

Time for an intervention!

CHAPTER TWO

A Lesson From Dad

"To lengthen thy life, lessen thy meals."

— Benjamin Franklin

My father was a hard-working Wisconsin cheesemaker-turned-dentist who struggled with weight gain for as long as I could remember.

Hours spent bent over his patients in the dental chair made for a pretty sedentary lifestyle, and the extra pounds began to add up over the years.

I remember how he would complain about the lack of time in life. He wanted to spend time with his six children and wife while eating right to stay healthy, but he also had to maintain a successful dental practice to support his family.

In an attempt to gain control of his weight, Dad signed up all the able-bodied males in the family with a membership to the YMCA. In theory, we were to hit the gym every Saturday morning as a family.

Despite all the activities offered such as weight training, the sauna, the pool, basketball, etc., the best part of going to the Y was our new addiction to the snack shop which had a tempting variety of food and drinks (Coke, Mountain Dew, prepackaged cheeseburgers to heat in the microwave, chips, and candy galore).

Dad's plan was a good one. **But instead of losing weight with our gym membership, we all GAINED weight, including dear old Dad.**

Pretty soon the gym membership went by the wayside, and my brothers and I joined school wrestling and football teams. Dad watched Watergate on the television with a Tab cola by his side when he wasn't attending our games.

Determined to address his weight gain, Dad began a medical fact-based calorie restriction diet. It was quite a program, as Dad claimed that a reduction in calories resulted in weight loss.

Dad religiously weighed his food to measure his calorie intake on a daily basis, and this program worked wonders for him. He was able to get back to a healthy weight, and he soon felt as good as he did in his thinner days.

He made a strong commitment to stay trim for the rest of his life. And he kept it!

For me, this was the "a-ha" moment in Dad's story: losing weight for him was all about restricting calories, not exercise or fads!

Some of the best advice my father gave me later on was:

The ability to maintain discipline and to appreciate your body as a gift from God shows respect for yourself and God. By maintaining your body through proper eating and caloric management, not exercise, you can go to work energetically and provide for your family.

Wow! How is that for a life lesson?

You can see part of why I had been so frustrated when I continued to gain weight despite all my efforts. My father's words rang true in my ears, yet before discovering the beauty of fasting, I hadn't been able to find the success he did.

The reason the diet worked for my father was the strict restriction of calories. He was willing to put in the time and effort to count every calorie and weigh his food for every meal, snack, and piece of cheese.

I wasn't.

Dad taught me that restricting calories is the primary method to achieve weight control. Exercise is critical to health but should be secondary when trying to lose weight.

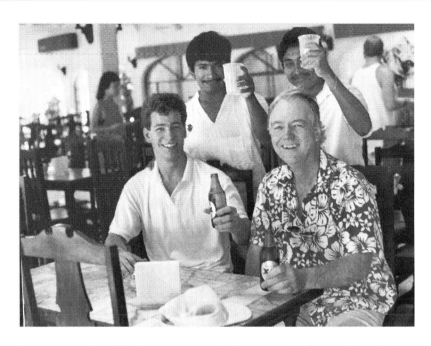

With Dad – getting the life lesson on weight control through calorie restriction.

CHAPTER THREE

A Year in a Life

"After ten years of a seemingly minor 1.85-pound weight gain per year, you will be at least 15 pounds overweight. In 20 years: Houston, we have a problem."

— Johnny Z

If you dare, face the fact that Americans who experience weight gain over 20 years from age 30 to 50 with an increase of 1.85 pounds per year will gain THIRTY POUNDS.

Believe it or not, that's quite a conservative estimate.

According to the Center for Disease Control and Prevention, the statistics are even worse:

- Percent of adults aged 20 and over with obesity: 37.9% (2013–2014)

- Percent of adults aged 20 and over who are overweight, including obese: 70.7% (2013–2014)

- Percent of adolescents aged 12–19 years with obesity: 20.6% (2013–2014)

- Percent of children aged 6–11 years with obesity: 17.4% (2013–2014)

- Percent of children aged 2–5 years with obesity: 9.4% (2013–2014)

Want to know what our friends at the CDC say about the consequences of obesity?

People who have obesity, compared to those with an average or healthy weight, are at increased risk for serious disease and health conditions, including the following:

- All–causes of death (mortality)

- Coronary heart disease

- Stroke

- Gallbladder disease

- Osteoarthritis (a breakdown of cartilage and bone within a joint)

- Sleep apnea and breathing problems

- Some cancers (endometrial, breast, colon, kidney, gallbladder, and liver)

- High blood pressure (Hypertension)

- High LDL cholesterol, low HDL cholesterol, or high levels of triglycerides (Dyslipidemia)

- Type 2 diabetes

- Low quality of life

- Mental illness such as clinical depression, anxiety, and other mental disorders
- Body pain and difficulty with physical functioning

No way, José! That's not gonna be me.

I worked too hard climbing the ladder at the office and raising three beautiful girls just to get fat and check out early due to one of the above!

But I was so curious to know how this weight gain happens so easily?

I mean, I have kids to keep up with!

I invite you to take a look at a year of my life and see if you can relate. I estimate:

- 360 dinners
- 101 big lunches
- 790 cocktails
- 65 desserts
- 71 small bags of chips
- 105 dedicated workouts
- Said no to french fries 100 times
- Declined a second helping 41 times
- Said yes to a "small" second helping 82 times
- Gave up most desserts and cream sauces
- Went to 17 killer barbecues

- Chowed down at five "pancake breakfasts" (because who can say *no* to the Boy Scouts?)
- Did I mention the Girl Scout cookies?

There is the long slide into the holidays starting with Thanksgiving dinner, followed by weeks of Christmas parties and eggnog (I love it), cocktails, and lots of home-cooked deliciousness.

In-laws and friends begged me to take a second helping. *"We're not going to eat it, so you have to!"* Plus, the always classic, *"Don't let it go to waste, Johnny!"*

There were vacations where I ate whatever I wanted because, "I am on vacation, for Pete's sake! Nobody diets on vacation!"

There were hot dogs, cheese fries, Super Bowl parties, and extra helpings of warm bread with butter whenever I stumbled upon that sitting on the table.

Let's not forget the hours and hours spent at my job behind a desk, sitting in an airplane flying to or from my office, or behind the wheel of a car.

THAT WHOLE YEAR boils down to a small 1.85-pound weight gain by New Year's Day. On the surface, it doesn't sound too bad, 1.85 pounds. That's not much, right?

But that gain repeats itself year after year until ten years pass and you're 18 pounds heavier without even realizing it was happening.

WEIGHT GAIN ONLY 1.85 lbs/Year		
AGE	WEIGHT	TOTAL Lbs
35	155.00	Start
36	156.85	1.85
37	158.70	3.70
38	160.55	5.55
39	162.40	7.40
40	164.25	9.25
41	166.10	11.10
42	167.95	12.95
43	169.80	14.80
44	171.65	16.65
45	173.50	18.50
18.5 POUNDS in 10 YEARS		

Take a look at the chart to see how easily this happens to the majority of Americans who experience a "minor" weight gain of 1.5 to 2 pounds a year. Obesity creeps in on cat's feet, as they say.

With this gradual weight gain, you find yourself at risk for the CDC's handy little list of *The Consequences of Obesity* I referenced above.

The damage from carrying extra weight is well documented. You don't need me to tell you that. You can look around and see the evidence of health problems associated with obesity.

So many diets are available to aid in weight loss and weight management and yet Americans are still fat and overweight. It's clear these diets don't work, as the obesity epidemic continues to grow in our country.

Whether it's a dislike of the foods in the various plans, problems applying the plans to a busy personal schedule, or that the diets are too complex, too slow, or too expensive, it's a fact that diets are not working for Americans.

Unless you're paying attention and taking action as soon as you notice that extra pound, you'll find yourself on the bus to obesity. This onset of weight is impossible to halt without dedicated attention to the scale and immediate action.

(Don't worry, I'm going to show you exactly what to do when I explain the Z-FAST.)

TIPPING THE SCALE

Most Americans don't bother to look ten years into the future, and probably not 35 years ahead to understand that there is a cumulative math equation going on here.

Your weight is a balancing act, but the equation is simple, undeniable, and unavoidable:

If you eat more calories than you burn, you gain weight.

Every 3,500 calories of extra food you eat will add one pound of FAT.

Yikes!

Even a small extra amount or indulgence of calories builds over time to added weight, slowly but surely!

Extra Intake per Week	
One large glass of wine	200 calories
One cranberry muffin	400 calories
One glass of orange juice	200 calories
Extra Calories/Week Total	800 calories

For example, a normal daily intake is considered to be 2,500 calories for a 180-pound human.

Let's say ONCE A WEEK you drank one extra glass of wine, a glass of orange juice, and you ate one cranberry muffin.

Those 800 calories per week × 52 weeks = 41,600,000 calories/3,500 (one pound) = 12 pounds weight gain in a single year.

That's 48 pounds over four years!

Now that's not exactly gorging yourself, as it's only three small extra items in an entire week.

But you can see how quickly the calories add up.

The equation is unavoidable: If you eat more calories than you burn, you gain weight.

Conversely, if you eat fewer calories than you burn, you lose weight.

Folks, this isn't "fake" math. It's a fact!

Because 3,500 calories equal one pound (0.45 kilogram) of fat, you would need to burn (use up) 3,500 calories to lose one single pound.

You can lose all those extra weekly calories by fasting one day.

A full fasting day (no food) equaling about 32 hours will draw down from your fat reserves about 3,000 calories.

Z-FASTING allows you to lose any extra weight you already have, plus stop that incremental yearly weight gain in the years that follow.

It's easy math!

Make a lifetime commitment NOW to your ideal weight so that by the end of each year you won't ever again experience that 1.85-pound gain!

And if we are honest, that annual weight gain is not 1.85 pounds a year. It's more like five pounds.

That'll put you at fifteen pounds of extra unwanted weight in just three short years.

That's why I designed Z-FAST — a new health revolution that will keep you off the CDC's statistic list!

CHAPTER FOUR

The Truth Revealed in Science: Fasting is Good for You

"Our genetic heritage is not used to stocked fridges, constant feeding, and ready-to-eat super-high-caloric meals all day long."

— Johnny Z

Okay, I hear you.

"Johnny Z, why would you want to go through what must be that uncomfortable feeling of not eating for an entire day?"

Why would you do that to yourself?

Surely you can find some other way to maintain your weight?

I mean, there's always liposuction and lap-band surgery, right?

WRONG.

(Well I mean, yes, those invasive procedures exist — but they are not solutions for most of us!)

Even if you would go so far as to have surgery or liposuction, without permanently changing your way of eating, that insidious weight gain we discussed will happen again.

And again. And again.

There's no way around it, folks!

You'll gain three to five pounds a quarter — or 1.85 to 12 pounds a year!

Surgery of any kind is tough on the body. (Plus, it's expensive!)

And dieting for the rest of your life would be well, frankly, ANNOYING.

Who wants to do that?

Who wants to be that guy or gal at the party talking about their diet and what he or she can and can't eat?

NOT ME, MAN.

I like having friends.

The reason why intermittent fasting is such an obvious choice is that IT'S GOOD FOR YOU!

There's no downside (other than a limited amount of hunger – and you already know that when you feel that hunger kick in, it means some fat-burning is going on).

The Z-FAST method is an eating pattern where you cycle between periods of eating and fasting.

Intermittent Fasting Health Advantages

Z-FAST
Intermittent Fasting Health Advantages

1 — Weight Loss
2 — Metabolic Rate Boost
3 — Burns Fat First
4 — Human Growth Hormone
5 — Physiological Power Over Constant Feeding
6 — Improve Insulin Levels
7 — Improve Heart Health – Clogged Arteries
8 — Live Longer

Not only does this establish a weight-loss pattern, but numerous studies show that it can have powerful benefits for your body and brain.

Check out the evidence-based health benefits of the Z-FAST!

If you think that this whole fasting thing is a little nuts, let me tell you, the idea of fasting is nothing crazy!

I mean, you do it every night when you're sleeping, which is the essential time for the body to restore optimal health.

Fasting allows your body to reprogram and heal as it switches from burning glucose from eating to burning fat to get the energy it needs.

Check out the movie *The Science of Fasting* produced by Sylvain Gilman and Thierry de Lestrade. It gives a fascinating peek into how clinics in Russia and Germany treat chronic illnesses such as asthma, hypertension, and obesity through MEDICAL fasts that can last as many as 12 to 14 days.

Even more surprising is that fasting is an accepted part of public health policy in some countries!

- Twelve public hospitals in Germany have an entire floor dedicated to fasting patients!

- The Buchinger Wilhelmi Clinic in Überlingen, Germany treats patients for rheumatism, rheumatoid arthritis, diabetes, and hypertension with a fasting regime.

□ The Goryachinsk Sanatorium claims that two-thirds of their patients see improvements after one or two fasting sessions.

□ And at the Moscow Psychiatric Institute, doctors have found that fasting has a stimulant and antidepressant effect.

It should be noted that the Mayo Clinic has advised that, "There are concerns about the potential side effects of regular fasting for certain people or in specific circumstances:

- People with eating disorders may end up binge eating more after fasting.

- Fasting and exercising at the same time may lead to low blood sugar (hypoglycemia), which can cause dizziness, confusion, and lightheadedness.

- Fasting by people taking diabetes medications can lead to severe hypoglycemia and can lead to serious health issues."

If you have a medical condition or health concern, please see your physician before beginning any health regimen such as the intermittent fasting methods discussed in this book.

CHAPTER FIVE

So How Does Fasting Work in the Human Body?

"A little starvation can really do more for the average sick man than can the best medicines and the best doctors."

— Mark Twain

First, understand that the body uses three fuels for power:

❶ Glucose (direct energy from meals to the bloodstream)

❷ Lipids (stored fats)

❸ Protein (which is converted to glucose)

Fasting causes a state of stress in the body which activates recovery mechanisms—the kind that is mostly inactive due to the Western lifestyle of never skipping a meal!

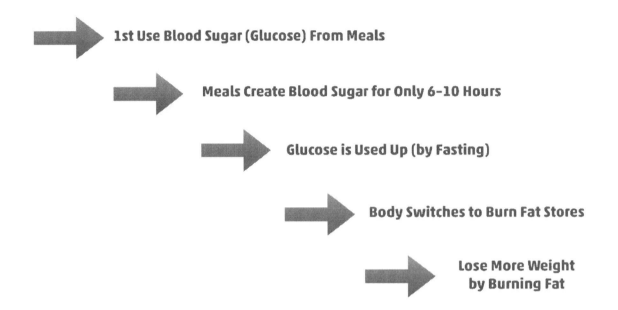

ENERGY SOURCE: Fasting Switches Body to Burn Fat Stores

➡ 1st Use Blood Sugar (Glucose) From Meals

➡ Meals Create Blood Sugar for Only 6-10 Hours

➡ Glucose is Used Up (by Fasting)

➡ Body Switches to Burn Fat Stores

➡ Lose More Weight by Burning Fat

Let's look at what happens in the body during a fast:

- The body senses starvation after 6–8 hours
- An alert is sent
- Hormones mobilize in the body
- HGH rises
- Metabolism increases
- Fat burning machine is turned on
- Reserves are tapped into (otherwise known as FAT!)
- An anti-inflammatory effect begins to heal the body

- Blood glucose levels normalize

- Blood pressure drops

Our evolution involved regular fasting as our ancestors had to find food. Our lifestyle of easily available food is the anomaly!

The body is better equipped to go without food from time to time than it is to be fed without a fast.

Some believe that fasting slows the metabolism and that you need to eat five meals a day to keep your body from thinking it should hold on to fat.

NOT TRUE.

Unlike how our ancestors lived, if you're continually feeding your body, it will never burn the fat stores around your belly. It won't have to, because it takes an average of five hours to burn off a meal.

During periods of fasting, your body will need to get energy after burning through a meal's worth of available glucose.

Where does it look for fuel? In those fat stores, otherwise known as belly fat, bottom fat, and neck fat.

Fasting works on both sides of the weight loss equation:

❶ **Caloric intake is lowered, and**

❷ **The process of burning fat is accelerated.**

The latest breakthrough studies have shown that metabolism goes up 3–14% during fasting.[5] This is part of the bodily process where you can jumpstart metabolism to get a short-term win without dieting every day for 30 long days.

Periodic fasts are way better, shorter, and deliver health benefits along the way!

All this for just not eating for half a day or a full day?

YES.

Once again, I ask: Who wants to suffer from limited portions, specific types of food, the cabbage diet, the Zone, and go through pain for extended weeks only to gain it back?

NOT ME.

Read on!

---

[5] "10 Evidence-Based Health Benefits of Intermittent Fasting." *Healthline*, Healthline Media,
  www.healthline.com/nutrition/10-health-benefits-of-intermittent-fasting

CHAPTER SIX

Fasting and the Heart

"Fasting is the greatest remedy, the physician within."

— Paracelsus

First, let's talk statistics.

According to the Centers for Disease Control and Prevention:

- About 610,000 people die of heart disease in the United States every year — that's one in every four deaths.

- Heart disease is the leading cause of death for both men and women.

- Coronary heart disease (CHD) is the most common type of heart disease, killing over 370,000 people annually.

WHOA!

If that isn't enough to inspire you to do whatever you can to prevent yourself from becoming a statistic, I don't know what is.

Luckily for us fasters, the folks at the University of Utah discovered that people fasting for just one day a month were 40 percent less likely to suffer from clogged arteries.

They also discovered that short daily fasts (for 12–16 hours, which would be skipping breakfast or dinner) or a once–per–week daily fast could have health benefits.[6]

Dr. Haitham Ahmed is a cardiologist at the famous Cleveland Clinic in Ohio. He says research is showing that fasting can help lower blood pressure, reduce cholesterol, control diabetes, and reduce weight. He advises that eating less, in general, is better, but fasting for short periods offers distinct advantages for the heart.

"Four of the **major risks for heart disease are high blood pressure and cholesterol, diabetes and weight**, so there's a secondary impact," Dr. Ahmed says. "If we reduce those [high numbers], we can reduce the risk of heart disease."

Dr. Ahmed isn't the only physician who is a fan of fasting.

The Mayo Clinic's Dr. Francisco Lopez-Jimenez claims, "At least one study has indicated that people who follow a fasting diet may have better heart health than people who don't." He says this may be due to the idea that people who routinely fast have self-control, and that this behavior may translate into weight control and better eating choices when they aren't fasting.

---

[6] "Fasting diet: Can it improve my heart health?" Mayo Clinic, Mayo Foundation for Medical Education and Research, 28 Sept. 2017, www.mayoclinic.org/diseases-conditions/heart-disease/expert-answers/fasting-diet/faq-20058334

Regular fasting and better heart health may also be linked to the way the body metabolizes cholesterol and sugar. Controlling both of these can reduce the risk of weight gain and the potential to develop diabetes, two known risk factors for heart disease.

Regular fasting can also decrease low-density lipoprotein, or "bad," cholesterol. Fasting has gained significant scientific and medical acceptance.

Don't want to become a statistic?

Turn the page!

CHAPTER SEVEN

Fasting and Cell, Gene, and Hormone Function

"In a fast, the body tears down its defective parts and then builds anew when eating is resumed."

— Herbert M. Shelton

Intermittent fasting works on both sides of the caloric equation by boosting the metabolic rate (calories out) and reducing the amount of food eaten (calories in).

Short-term fasting has been shown to increase metabolic rate by 3.6%–14%, helping you burn even more calories.

During periods of fasting, the body benefits from a slew of hormonal changes:

- Insulin levels drop.
- Human growth hormone (HGH) increases.

- Cells initiate crucial cellular repair processes and change which genes they express.

- Lowered insulin and higher HGH levels, along with increased amounts of norepinephrine (noradrenaline) speed up the breakdown of body fat and facilitate its use for needed energy.

One of the main benefits of fasting comes from reducing insulin, which improves heart health, but luckily for you, there are many more benefits!

GROWING THAT HGH

Counter-regulatory hormones are increased during periods of fasting such as noradrenalin, cortisol, and HGH.

These guys increase blood glucose when food is not arriving to provide it.

Around 4 a.m. every morning, your body experiences a counter-regulatory surge as it prepares itself to get up and run.

This includes a shot of HGH so you awake refreshed with the energy to begin the day.

HGH has a rather short lifespan (just a few minutes at most) as the body secretes it in short bursts, so we don't become resistant to it.

HGH heads straight to the liver, where it is metabolized into other growth hormones.

The backstory on HGH is that it causes kids to grow, so that's important of course. We peak at puberty, and then HGH levels steadily decline as we age.

Low levels of HGH in adults tend to result in excess body fat, lower lean body mass, and decreased bone mass.

"But, Johnny Z, if lower levels of HGH result in increased fat and decreased body mass, why can't we just supplement HGH artificially?"

Well, it's available and has been shown to get results (a loss of fat and an increase in muscle mass just like fasting). The problem is that it isn't achieved naturally and results in a few pesky side-effects: increased blood pressure, higher blood sugars, fluid retention, increase of pre-diabetes, and enlarged heart.[7]

Who needs that?

NO BUENO.

But another study involving increasing HGH through the natural means of fasting brought about entirely different side effects.

In 1982, Kerndt, Naughton, Driscoll & Loxterkamp published a study of a 40-day fast of a patient who decided to undergo the fast for religious purposes. Yes, 40 days!

His glucose and insulin levels dropped 80% while his HGH levels increased by 1,250% WITHOUT any of those pesky side effects.[8]

[7 & 8] "Fasting and growth hormone." *Diet Doctor*, 15 Dec. 2017,
www.dietdoctor.com/fasting-and-growth-hormone

No increased glucose.

No increased blood pressure.

All the benefits with none of the side effects!

BRING ON THE GHRELIN!
(THE HUNGRY STOMACH HORMONAL SMART BOOST)

Our bodies produce ghrelin to stimulate appetite when the stomach is empty. (As if we need to be reminded to eat!)

There is some pretty cool evidence out there that ghrelin enhances cognition![9]

(I know I certainly feel sharper on my fast days.)

The hungrier we are, the more ghrelin is secreted into the bloodstream.

Ghrelin is like an all-natural smart pill!

Jeffrey Davies at Swansea University, UK, and his team say ghrelin can stimulate brain cells to divide and multiply, a process called neurogenesis. Upon adding ghrelin to mouse brain cells grown in a

---

[9] "Hungry stomach hormone promotes growth of new brain cells." *New Scientist*,
www.newscientist.com/article/2128695-hungry-stomach-hormone-promotes-growth-of-new-brain-cells/

dish, "it switched on a gene known to trigger neurogenesis, called fibroblast growth factor."

Voilà, fresh new brain cells!

So, it follows that fasting causes your body to secrete ghrelin, which stimulates cognition. That's why I feel sharper on fasting days even though I have not eaten.

Makes a lot of sense if you THINK about it. (Pun intended.)

The caveman needed to become sharper when he was hungry so that he could find food. If he were to become weaker in times of hunger, his chances of feeding himself would drop tremendously, right?

Ghrelin has been found to be at lower levels in folks suffering from Parkinson's disease.

Davies' team discovered that when brain cells in a dish were encouraged to mimic Parkinson's, adding ghrelin to the mix kept them from dying ...

I could stop writing right here.

If you've ever dealt with a family member suffering from dementia, you understand how important it is to keep your mind in tip-top shape.

FASTING AND INSULIN

Ingesting foods raises insulin levels, which of course we need in reasonable doses or we wouldn't be able to function.

To lower insulin, you deny the body food (for a period).

The body needs to keep functioning without food, so it will find ways to maintain blood glucose levels, which means turning to stored fats.

The benefits of lowering insulin are many.

Since we have become a country of eaters, we have trained our bodies to rely on the regular delivery of sugar. But we rarely turn to burning stored fat for energy.

The result is Type 2 diabetes has become way too common in recent decades.

While middle-aged and older adults are still at the highest risk of developing Type 2 diabetes, our friends at the CDC say Type 2 diabetes in younger people is on the rise.

According to the CDC, there were a total of 1.7 million new diabetes cases in 2012.

In 2012, adults aged 45 to 64 were the most diagnosed age group with diabetes. New cases of both Type 1 and Type 2 diabetes in people aged 20 years and older were distributed as follows:

- Ages 20 to 44: 371,000 new cases

- Ages 45 to 64: 892,000 new cases

- Age 65 and older: 400,000 new cases

People aged 45 to 64 were also developing diabetes at a faster rate, edging out adults aged 65 and older.

Interestingly, intermittent fasting has been shown to have significant benefits for insulin resistance and leads to a reduction in blood sugar levels. Studies on intermittent fasting show fasting blood sugar and fasting insulin have been reduced.

The natural conclusion is that intermittent fasting may be highly protective for people who are at risk of developing Type 2 diabetes.

FASTING AND INFLAMMATION AND OXIDATIVE STRESS IN THE BODY

Researchers at Yale School of Medicine discovered that β-hydroxybutyrate (BHB), which is produced by the body in response to dieting or fasting, directly inhibits NLRP3, which is part of a complex set of proteins called the inflammasome.

Too sciencey for you?

I get it.

Let me break this down, because I get it that not everyone's the science geek that I am:

Fasting causes the body to produce a cool little hormone called BHB, which inhibits proteins that cause inflammation.

This is darn good news for those suffering from autoimmune diseases such as Type 2 diabetes, Alzheimer's disease, atherosclerosis, and other autoinflammatory disorders.

Vishwa Deep Dixit, one of the researchers and professors in the Section of Comparative Medicine at Yale School of Medicine, stresses the importance of BHB's role in fighting inflammation.

BHB is produced by the body in response to fasting, high-intensity exercise, caloric restriction, or consumption of the low-carbohydrate ketogenic diet.

Dixit says, "It is well known that fasting and calorie restriction **reduces inflammation in the body**, but it was unclear how immune cells adapt to reduced availability of glucose and if they can respond to metabolites produced from fat oxidation."

You've heard of those pesky free radicals, right?

Well, apparently they run roughshod over the body, damaging important stuff like protein and DNA.

Free radicals are a part of oxidative stress, which is one of the steps towards aging and other diseases.

Several studies show that intermittent fasting may enhance the body's resistance to oxidative stress, thereby naturally combating free radicals.

FASTING AND CELLULAR REPAIR PROCESSES

Your cells get busy during fasting.

There's this scary-sounding process your body undergoes called autophagy, or "self-eating."

Uh, what?

In other words, the body cannibalizes itself.

But wait, that's a good thing, as the cells consume tissue during a metabolic process occurring in the fasting state, and certain diseases.

The body creates membranes to hunt the dead, diseased, or worn-out cells, and then recycle them to make new cell parts.

This is your very own cellular "waste removal" process!

These cells break down and metabolize broken and dysfunctional proteins that build up inside them.

They "clean house" if you will.

This metabolic path clears the way for all the junk material in the cells to be moved out.

FASTING AND THE PREVENTION OF CANCER

While this is a vast subject, I'll summarize what I've learned not only about fasting's role in the prevention of cancer but how fasting improves the chemotherapy experience for some patients.

Significant research needs to be done here to provide necessary medical guidance.

Valter Longo (who can be seen in the movie *The Science of Fasting*), professor and director of the USC Longevity Institute at the USC Leonard Davis School of Gerontology, has led a couple of studies on the effects of fasting on cancer and chemotherapy.

One study showed that a "fasting-like diet with chemotherapy strips away the guard that protects breast cancer and skin cancer cells from the immune system."

Say what?

When fasting during chemotherapy, cancer cells are less protected, therefore more vulnerable to treatment!

According to Professor Longo, "The mouse study on skin and breast cancers is the first study to show that a diet that mimics fasting may activate the immune system and expose the cancer cells to the immune system. This could be a very inexpensive way to make a wide range of cancer cells more vulnerable to an attack by the immune cells while also making cancer more sensitive to the chemotherapy."[10]

Fasting revs up the immune system, making cancer cells more vulnerable to the effects of chemo.

---

[10] "Fasting-like diet turns the immune system against cancer." *USC News*, 5 Feb. 2018, news.usc.edu/103972/fasting-like-diet-turns-the-immune-system-against-cancer/

These studies are building upon earlier research that shows that fasting-type diets "starve" cancer cells, allowing chemotherapy to better target the cells.

This response in the immune system may be an evolved mechanism to protect us from the disease.

"It may be that by always being exposed to so much food, we are no longer taking advantage of natural protective systems which allow the body to kill cancer cells. But by undergoing a fasting-mimicking diet, you can let the body use sophisticated mechanisms able to identify and destroy the bad but not good cells in a natural way," Professor Longo said.

FASTING AND THE BRAIN

We sure know those excess calories aren't good for the belly, but we're learning they're not good for the brain either.

Z-FAST to the rescue!

Neuroscientist Matt Mattson's studies have shown that reducing energy intake by fasting several days a week might help the brain avoid neurodegenerative diseases like Alzheimer's and Parkinson's.[11]

This is a big deal.

---

[11] Mattson, M P, et al. "Meal size and frequency affect neuronal plasticity and vulnerability to disease: cellular and molecular mechanisms." *Journal of Neurochemistry*, U.S. National Library of Medicine, Feb. 2003, www.ncbi.nlm.nih.gov/pubmed/12558961

(Remember that people with Parkinson's are found to have lower levels of HGH — which is increased tremendously during periods of fasting!)

Mattson claims fasting improves neural connections while protecting neurons against the accumulation of amyloid plaques, a protein found to be prevalent in people with Alzheimer's disease.

"Fasting is a challenge to your brain, and we think that your brain reacts by activating adaptive stress responses that help it cope with disease," says Mattson. "From an evolutionary perspective, it makes sense your brain should be functioning well when you haven't been able to obtain food for a while."

Remember my caveman analogy?

He had to be extra sharp to think about how to get food while fasting and hungry!

(That meat wasn't gonna cook itself!)

Several studies in rats have shown that intermittent fasting may increase the growth of new nerve cells, which should have benefits for brain function.

Fasting has also been shown to increase levels of the brain hormone called brain-derived neurotrophic factor (BDNF).

This all boils down to a simple fact: fasting stresses the brain, which causes the brain to fortify itself and reduce vulnerability to disease.

Intermittent fasting creates a cellular stress response that stimulates the production of proteins that enhance neuronal plasticity and resistance to oxidative and metabolic insults.

Fasting shocks the brain into creating new cells.

Not bad, huh?

FASTING AND A LONGER LIFE

There are a couple of main points tying fasting and lengthened lifespan together.

Lowered insulin during fasting seems to be one of the most important contributors to extending life.

As I mentioned earlier, insulin drops during a period of fasting.

The body dials back a bit and enters a conservation mode.

When you resume eating, your body is subsequently more sensitive to insulin.

This is kind of a big deal.

See, longer-living animals and people tend to have lower insulin levels in general. The thinking is that because their cells are more sensitive to insulin, they need less of it.

In comparison, the obese tend to have higher insulin levels, which is linked to diabetes and heart failure, which, as we read earlier, lead to heart disease and ultimately, death.[12]

---

[12] Haridy, Rich. "Harvard study uncovers why fasting can lead to a longer and healthier life." New Technology & Science News, *New Atlas*, 6 Nov. 2017, newatlas.com/fasting-increase-lifespan-mitochondria-harvard/52058/

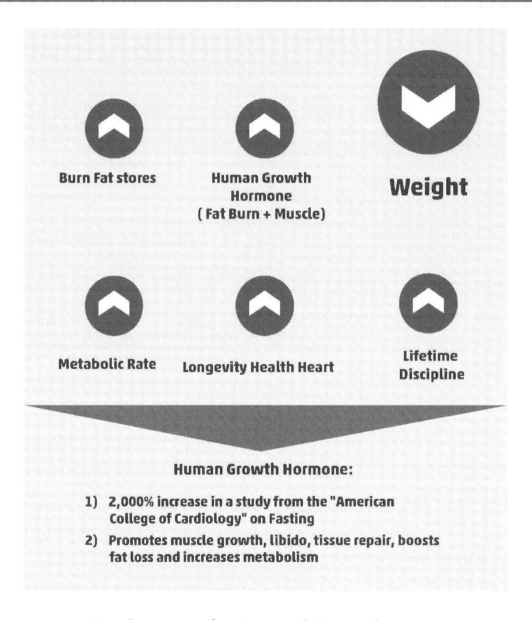

Intermittent Fast Advantages

Burn Fat stores

Human Growth Hormone (Fat Burn + Muscle)

Weight

Metabolic Rate

Longevity Health Heart

Lifetime Discipline

Human Growth Hormone:

1) 2,000% increase in a study from the "American College of Cardiology" on Fasting
2) Promotes muscle growth, libido, tissue repair, boosts fat loss and increases metabolism

The connection between fasting and living longer is continually being studied, but a promising new Harvard study is showing how fasting extends lifespan, retards aging and improves health.

"Low-energy conditions such as dietary restriction and intermittent fasting have previously been shown to promote healthy aging," explains Heather Weir, lead author of the study.

Their findings explained the "why" of it, showing that fasting manipulates "mitochondrial networks" in our cells to keep them youthful.

Researchers explain that mitochondria are "tiny little power plants" inside our cells and they have been found to be tied to cell aging.

Changing their shape can alter the length of life because it's when they get "stuck" that aging occurs.

Think of this little benefit, as *yoga for the cells!*

Keep them flexible, and you just might live longer.

CHAPTER EIGHT

Fasting Beats Exercise for Weight Loss: But Don't Stop Working Out

> "It's pretty easy to get people to eat 1,000 calories less per day, but to get them to do 1,000 calories per day of exercise — walking 10 miles — is daunting at many levels."
>
> — Michael Joyner, Mayo Clinic

First of all, YES, it's possible to work out while fasting.

NO, you won't feel weak and worthless.

On the contrary, if you can work out on FASTING days, the fat burn and muscle build are significantly boosted versus standard workouts.

Increased noradrenalin from fasting will allow you to train harder. At the same time, the elevated HGH stimulated by fasting increases muscle mass and makes a recovery from a workout easier and faster.

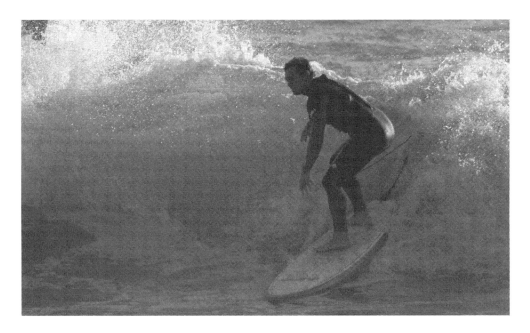

Johnny Z surfing on a full fast day. Getting the fasting triple burn – no calorie intake, a surge in fat storage burn, and exercise boosting the fat storage burn even more!

The folks who say fasting reduces muscle mass are uninformed. The opposite is true!

As I shared earlier, I have a degree in biology, so it was vital for me to see the best way to lose weight from a scientific perspective.

I also had to understand the role played by calories versus exercise.

Let's back up for a minute to review the math of weight loss.

Your weight is a balancing act, and caloric intake plays a significant role. Despite all the diet strategies out there, weight management still comes down to a simple math equation:

You must take in fewer calories than what you burn; there is no way around this fact!

It is likewise a fact that 3,500 calories from any food source equal one pound of human weight.

If you want to lose a pound, you must create a 3,500-calorie deficit.

That holds true whether you're 6' and 230 pounds, or you're 5' and 100 pounds: the math doesn't change.

Fad diets may promise that avoiding carbs or eating a mountain of grapefruit is the secret to weight loss.

Don't believe the hype.

"Exercise for weight loss is highly overrated," says Marc Reitman, chief of the diabetes, endocrinology and obesity branch of the National Institute of Diabetes and Digestive and Kidney Diseases, or NIDDK. "I think it's really great for being healthy, but I'm a strong believer that overeating is what causes obesity. To exercise your way out of overeating is impossible."

Put simply ...

You can't outrun a pizza!

CALORIES ARE FUEL FOR YOUR BODY

Calories are the energy of food.

Your body has a constant demand for energy and uses the calories to fuel your every action, from thinking to fidgeting to running a marathon.

How do we get calories?

Carbohydrates, fats, and proteins are the types of nutrients that contain calories and are the main energy sources for your body. Regardless of where they come from, the calories you eat are either converted to physical energy or stored in your body as fat.

These stored calories will remain in your body as fat unless you use them up, either by reducing calorie intake so that your body must draw on reserves for energy (stored fat) or by increasing physical daily activity so that you burn more calories than you take in.

No doubt you've heard that exercise is terrific and can solve weight issues.

"But can't I just run around the block a couple of times, Johnny Z?"

Well, sure you can.

But you're not going to lose much weight.

And if you want to lose weight, you're going to have to run around *quite a few blocks*.

Exercise is terrific.

No argument from me there.

We should all be exercising.

I surf two times a week and enjoy the heck out of it.

I also hike whenever I get the chance.

But exercising strictly for weight loss is not as effective as other methods, particularly fasting.

Michael Joyner, a Mayo Clinic researcher who studies how people respond to the stress of exercise, agrees. "The key for weight loss is to generate and maintain a calorie deficit," he says. "It's pretty easy to get people to eat 1,000 calories less per day, but to get them to do 1,000 calories per day of exercise — walking 10 miles — is daunting at many levels, including time and motivation."

How Many Calories Are You Burning?

Syracuse University researchers measured the actual calorie burn of 12 men and 12 women while running and walking 1,600 meters (roughly a mile) on a treadmill.[13]

Result: The men burned an average of 124 calories while running, and just 88 while walking. The women burned 105 and 74.

In theory, this sounds great.

If you're an average guy and you run five miles, you've burned off 5 × 124 calories = 620 calories. If you run two miles, you've burned off 2 × 124 calories = 248 calories.

To avoid weight gain from a chocolate chip cookie or a bag of small chips ... you have to run two miles.

TWO MILES!

It's tough to exercise your way to skinny.

---

[13] "Energy Expenditure of Walking and Running," published in Medicine & Science in *Sports & Exercise*.

Exercise vs the Calorie
Calorie is King

3,500 Calories = 1 lb.
Approximate Calories Burned by Activity
Example: Male, age 55, 5'11" 185 lbs

Activity	30 Minutes	40 minutes	# of 30-min sessions to lose 1 lb.	# of 60-min sessions to lose 1 lb.
Lifting Weights	144	192	24	12
Walking (4 mph)	216	289	16	8
Swimming (moderate)	255	340	14	7
Elliptical	477	636	7	4
Rowing (moderate)	294	392	12	6
Running Treadmill	250	350	14	7
Volleyball (recreation)	144	192	24	12
Surfing	128	170	27	14
Basketball (full court)	461	614	8	4
Skiing (downhill)	366	488	10	5
Dancing	344	459	10	5
Golfing	144	192	24	12

I don't know about you, but I'd rather enjoy my life.

Losing weight is really about eating LESS.

Hence the Z-FAST!

Losing weight through exercise alone is a daunting task, and it's just not that effective.

An entire high-energy, brutal workout is immediately negated with a single slice of pizza.

BENEFITS OF WORKING OUT WHILE FASTING

Remember in the previous chapter when we learned that higher levels of HGH in adults result in less body fat, more lean body mass (muscle), and increased bone mass?

Fasting HGH increase allows you to benefit from the anti-aging properties of HGH without any of the problems of excessive HGH.

Since fasting BOOSTS HGH, it follows that when you're working out during your fast, you'll burn more body fat and fight the decrease of body mass and bone mass.

This provides a triple win for the FASTER, making getting ripped even easier.

Dr. Michael VanDerschelden, or Dr. Mike, as most people call him, is a Huntington Beach doctor who happens to be a nutrition and exercise expert. He is famous for implementing and mastering lifestyle changes like intermittent fasting combined with high intensity interval training which maximizes health and function.

In his book, *The Scientific Approach to Intermittent Fasting*, he discusses intermittent fasting, the Ketogenic diet and a direct approach to combining serious exercise with fasting. Dr. Mike has done a lot of research on fasting with exercise and scientifically lays out why he is a huge proponent of the practice and its benefits.

He maintains that if you're looking to be healthy, then you'll NEED to have adequate secretions of HGH (which I know you know by now is boosted by fasting).

The human body was made to not only survive but to thrive during regular blocks of fasting.

Once we entered the last 100 years of "three square meal" and "five small meals a day" thinking, everything changed.

We don't get the benefit of these hormone spikes as often as our ancestors did because we are eating all day long.

Dr. Mike says, "According to the American College of Cardiology, intermittent fasting triggers nearly a 1,300% increase in human growth hormone secretion in women and 2,000% increases in men. You're not able to get this from artificial injections, nothing. This is huge, and this is natural. Growth hormone is what keeps you healthy and younger; skin health, everything inside, lean muscle mass production, bone health, it's everything. Growth hormone is literally the key."[14]

---

[14] http://drkevinpecca.com/intermittent-fasting-and-the-ketogenic-diet-with-dr-mike-vanderschelden/

Many exercise enthusiasts and proponents of fasting have developed very innovative exercise protocols for building muscle mass and dropping pounds while fasting.

Mike Wilson, the fitness leader and owner of Cape May Fitness & Sports, is the Head Strength and Conditioning Coach. Along with Roberto Gonzalez (his medical science liaison with certificates in Biochemistry, Physiology, and Genetics from Harvard Medical School), they have come up with a popular and highly effective method for combining intermittent fasting with resistance training (weights).

"We see excellent results that can't be obtained with exercise alone. Fasting has changed my clients' lives and our professional approach to exercise programs," Mike says. His fasting and exercising seminars routinely sell out.

Most of Mike's clients don't want to exercise all the time to lose weight.

"They're very busy moms, and they want the weight loss. We have many clients having success in muscle building and fat reduction with fasting and exercise, including strength and fitness training. Doing high impact cross fit is great, and we train for that here, and maybe you can burn 500 calories. But that killer high-energy work out is canceled with one single piece of pizza. That's **why we now offer a combination course in FASTING along with a very specific exercise program** that can be a breakthrough for our clients."

Mike experiences very little effect on his energy level when he is fasting and working out. "My rule of thumb is to break my fast after my work out. I fast 20 hours, and then I work out. We advise breaking the fast with 20–50 grams of protein, such as four ounces of chicken breast or egg whites. Low carbs. After one hour you can add in other foods. You get a longer boost of fat burn that way."

It's important to keep in mind that the fat breakdown observed with increased HGH levels and the amount of fat lost is determined by the size of the caloric deficit (fasting plus exercise) and not by the increased amount of HGH secreted.

You are more likely to use stored fat as a fuel source when growth hormone is elevated — or when you are fasting!

Combining an exercise routine with a Z-FAST regimen makes sense for a variety of reasons.

Studies show that muscle does not spontaneously atrophy to a significant or even notable extent during an 18–20 hour FAST, contrary to what you may have heard.

You can rest assured that your hard-earned muscle will still be preserved! The body will only turn to muscle mass after it has run through all the fat stores.

As I've already mentioned, one of the scientific aspects of Intermittent Fasting is its potent influence on elevating HGH. This is healthy on its own, but when combined with exercise, the benefits are increased!

The primary purpose of HGH is to help break down stored fat, but it will not directly stimulate muscle growth or prevent muscle breakdown while in a calorie deficit.

The key takeaway here is that you are more likely to use stored fat as a fuel source when growth hormone is elevated — or when you are fasting.

I was highly interested in hearing that Cape May Fitness & Sports in New Jersey has been offering seminars in weight loss with intermittent fasting (Z-FAST's half-day fasting) combined with exercise protocols to its clients!

CHAPTER NINE

Religious Fasting

"My religion teaches me that whenever there is distress which one cannot remove, one must fast and pray."

— Gandhi

Nearly every culture in every country has practiced fasting, and in most cases, it's performed for religious reasons. The practice of fasting for religious purposes has been documented going back for millennia. The inconvenience of fasting is offered up for a greater cause which varies amongst the world's religions.

As a point of interest, highlighted below are the more familiar forms of religion, their fasting times, methods, and reasons for fasting.

Fasting Across Religions: a Pathway to Fasting

Religions	Fasting	Fasting Method	Reasons They Fast
Baha'i	During Ala, March 2-20 in the 19th month of the Baha'i year.	No food and drink from sunrise to sunset.month of the Baha'i year.	Fasting is for spiritual reasons and focus on their love for God.
Buddhist	For most types of Buddhism, fasting usually occurs on holidays and days with a full moon.	Usually means no solid food while some liquids are permitted.	Fasting is used for purification. The Theravadin and Tendai Buddhis monks fast to free the mind. Fasting is used to generate inner heat by some Tibetan Buddhist monks.
Catholic	On Ash Wednesday, Good Friday and all Fridays during the 40 days of Lent. In some parts of the world, people abstain from meat every Friday of the year.	Meat is forbidden on Ash Wednesday, Good Friday and all Fridays during Lent. Most Catholics give additional penance by abstaining from a particular favorite food, drink or activity during Lent.	Many reasons ranging from a form of discipline, to building solidarity with the unfortunate/ poor or a penance for sins. Fasting for Lent prepares the soul for the celebration of Easter when Jesus rose from the dead.
Eastern Orthodox	Lent, Apostles' Fast, Dormition Fast, the Nativity Fast, and several one-day fasts. Every Wednesday and Friday is considered a fast day (except those that fall during designated "fast-free weeks")	Prohibition of meat, eggs and dairy products. Fish is also prohibited on some fast days.	Exposes one to the grace of God and strengthens resistance to gluttony.
Hindu	On New Moon days and during festivals such as Shivaratri, Saraswati Puja, Durga Puja. In northern India, Women also fast on Karva Chauth.	For most, solid foods are eliminated with a periodic drink of water or milk. For others, it is a complete 24 hour fast of food or drink.	During mediation to enhance worship or concentration; as a form of sacrifice; and to purify oneself.
Jewish	The Day of Atonement called Yom Kippur as well as six other feast days on the Jewish calendar including the day the Jewish Temple was destroyed, Tisha B'Av.	From sundown to sundown, eating and drinking are forbidden on Yom Kippur and Tisha B'Av. Eating and drinking are forbidden only from sunrise to sundown on the other fast days.	As a means to make special requests to God and/or atonement for sins.
Mormon	Every first Sunday of the month. Fasting at will may also be practiced by some Individuals, families, or wards.	Abstaining from food and drink for two consecutive meals and donating food or money to the needy. After the fast, church members participate in a "fast and testimony meeting."	Closeness to God; concentration on God and religion. Individual or family fasts might be held to petition for a specific cause, such as healing for one who is sick or help with making a difficult decision.
Muslim	Ramadan, the ninth month of the Muslim calendar, which commemorates the period when the Qur'an was first revealed to the prophet Muhammad. Additionally, various Muslim customs recommend days and periods of fasting like every Monday or Thursday. Some muslims fast during the three days preceding Ramadan. Some fast during Sha'baan which is the month prior to Ramadan.	For the entire month of Ramadan, complete abstinence from food, drink, smoking, profane language, and sexual intercourse from before the break of dawn until sunset.	To emulate the prophet Muhammad who was said to fast.

Despite what can be considered varying beliefs among the world's religions, the motivations behind fasting were surprisingly similar:

- Atonement
- Discipline
- Enhance worship
- Devotion to God
- Penance
- Purification
- Resistance to gluttony

Fasting can't be all bad, huh?

It's interesting to think of fasting as a "spiritual weapon."

There are reasons that religions of all nations throughout history include the power of fasting.

And we know the ability to fast takes power, dedication, commitment, and strength!

The determination to temporarily give up earthly pleasures like food and drink shows a strong discipline in connecting to something bigger, something spiritual, and to live in a realm, if even for a short one day, that is not clouded by a constant, incessant gnawing to keep eating.

When fasting, you're temporarily disconnecting from the earthly rat race by practicing the discipline to say *no*.

Our maker has given each of us a beautiful temple: our body.

Let's honor it by keeping our weight in check!

Stop for a moment and consider how amazing our bodies are!

We need to manage our weight and respect our bodies as it will need to carry us, every day for 80+ years here on earth.

Fasting can help us connect to a higher level of respect for our bodies. The short-term pain we go through during fasting is a small trade-off that directly provides a healthy path to happiness.

Your body will love you.

THE PRACTICE OF FASTING IN CATHOLICISM

Being a Catholic, fasting or giving up something of value (usually something that you eat or drink) for 40 days is practiced in the Lenten period every year. It ends with Easter. I utilize the Lenten season as an extra reason to initiate the fast and allow for added focus.

I personally enjoy combining spirituality and health!

The Catholic Church has long espoused the importance of fasting in the life of every Christian; to practice self-denial to strengthen self-control and to enhance prayers. It is said in the gospels to "fast and pray" as they should go together as one event.

Fasting is the traditional way to deny the self, to put passions to death through fasting. Many Catholics also "give up" the pain of self-denial during a fast for a special intention or for a special purpose. This then can become a "fast and pray" special intention.

"Fasting" does not refer only to food (though it is most often practiced in this way), but also giving up what can be perceived as negative ways of being, such as gossiping, or criticizing others.

St. Francis de Sales recommends fasting to, "control greediness, and to keep the sensual appetites and the whole-body subject to the law of the Spirit."

But Catholics are warned that fasting is not the goal, but a tool in ascent toward becoming a better person and gaining a closer relationship with God: fasting is used to strengthen and cleanse the self.

As the *Lenten Triodion* says, "Let us set out with joy upon the season of the Fast and prepare ourselves for spiritual combat. Let us purify our soul and cleanse our flesh; and as we fast from food, let us abstain from every passion."

St. Basil the Great sums up many of the Catholic feelings on fasting and prayer: "Fasting is a good safeguard for the soul, a steadfast companion for the body. Fasting gives birth to prophets and strengthens the powerful; fasting makes lawgivers wise. Fasting is a weapon for the valiant, and a gymnasium for athletes. Fasting repels temptations, anoints unto piety; it is the comrade of watchfulness and the artificer of chastity. In war, it fights bravely, in peace it teaches stillness."

THE JEWISH TRADITION OF FASTING

In the Jewish religion, there are 25 different holidays and events (some lasting for days) associated with the tradition of fasting. Fasting is only required on Yom Kippur, beginning just before sundown on the first evening to darkness on the following evening when three stars can be seen in the sky.

The other holiday where fasting is required is Tisha B'Av.

Aside from abstaining from food, supplicants are not permitted to wash, wear leather, use scents such as colognes, or have sexual relations.

Most Jewish holidays that involve fasting are to observe death, destruction, or sieges.

Interestingly, fasting is called "self-affliction" in the Torah!

The Jewish people fast for several reasons, including atonement, mourning, supplication (to change God's mind or get His attention), in preparation for battle, for piety, on the anniversary of a parent's death.

An ancient custom exists whereby the bride and groom fast on the day of their wedding!

On Yom Kippur (Day of Atonement), God instructs the Jewish people, "You shall afflict your souls."

During the 24-hour fast, worshippers spend the entire day in prayer, practicing repentance, contrition, and introspection together. In a community environment, Jews chant the confession of sins, resulting in spiritual cleansing.

This denial of pleasure during a fast is offered as *teshuvah,* or repentance.

ISLAM AND FASTING

Fasting in Islam traditionally brings to mind the month of Ramadan. The holiday begins on the ninth month of the Islamic calendar when the crescent moon is sighted (although discrepancies have existed for some time) and ends 29–30 days later when the crescent moon is again in sight.

In Islam (which means surrendering to the will of God and making peace: *al-silm*), fasting is used for spiritual fulfillment. The thought is that a month of fasting will bring a multiplication of blessings.

The Prophet Mohammed reportedly said, "When the month of Ramadan starts, the gates of Heaven are opened, and the gates of Hell are closed, and the devils are chained."

Fasting allows Muslims to experience *tawhid*: perfection. The Quran teaches *tawhid*: "There is no deity (no one worth being loved and worshipped) saved He, to Him alone belong the attributes of perfection."

Therefore, when Muslims fast they can reflect on the many gifts bestowed upon humanity and can contemplate perfection, develop gratitude, and be aware of the needy nature of humanity.

This "neediness" is made evident through hunger, allowing Muslims to feel compassion for others and recognize that we all belong to the same maker.

While fasting from dawn until sunset, Muslims are expected to increase devotion and acts of charity while refraining from consuming food, drinking liquids, smoking, and engaging in sexual relations.

Like Catholics, Muslims are instructed to avoid the negative types of behaviors such as gossiping and lying.

Ramadan ends each evening usually breaking the fast with delicious dates (said to have been eaten by Muhammad), then prayers.

Family and friends often gather each evening to share a feast (called *iftar*) consisting of water, juices, dates, salads and appetizers, one or more main dishes, and various kinds of desserts to break their fast.

BUDDHISM AND FASTING

Fasting in Buddhism is a mixed bag.

Stories report that when Siddhārtha Gautama (who would become the Buddha) sought enlightenment, he fasted for several years eating only one sesame seed and one berry per day.

As his meditation did not progress, he decided that "the middle way" was best, and preached moderation in fasting from that point. He sat in meditation until he reached enlightenment.

It is also said that the Buddha spoke highly of fasting and noted during his fasts, "My soul becomes brighter, my spirit, more alive in wisdom and truth."

Buddhist monks and nuns today traditionally do not eat after their noon meal until sunrise of the next day, although this practice varies among the differing traditions.

It is thought that the Buddha's recommendation for fasting was for health reasons alone. He said, "I do not eat in the evening and thus am free from illness and affliction and enjoy health, strength, and ease." (M.I,473).

Fasting in Buddhism is now considered not to be around health, but discipline.

Self-discipline allows us to acquire self-control, which is believed to lead to the development of increased spirituality.

The Buddha underwent long periods of fasting during his learning period.

One described fast involved eating once every seven days or eating one fruit per day, resulting in emaciation.

However, it is believed that once he attained enlightenment, he did not fast nor recommend fasting.

Since his fasting experiences played a central role in the formation of Buddhism, his experiences set a fasting example for his followers making fast a part of Buddhism.

> **"Fasting is a good safeguard for the soul, a steadfast companion for the body. Fasting gives birth to prophets and strengthens the powerful."**
>
> **— St. Basil the Great**

CHAPTER TEN

Lifetime Commitment Weight

"Most dieters fail to keep off the weight they lose, and most gain back MORE THAN THEY LOST. There is little support for the notion that diets lead to lasting weight loss or health benefits."

— National Institute of Health

The first step of the Z-FAST is to determine your lifetime commitment weight.

This number is crucial because the most critical point of Z-FAST is that you promise yourself that you will never, ever go over your lifetime commitment weight, EVER, without immediate fasting intervention.

I suggest that you be reasonable with your number.

You might want to choose your high school weight, but don't be tempted to set yourself up for failure.

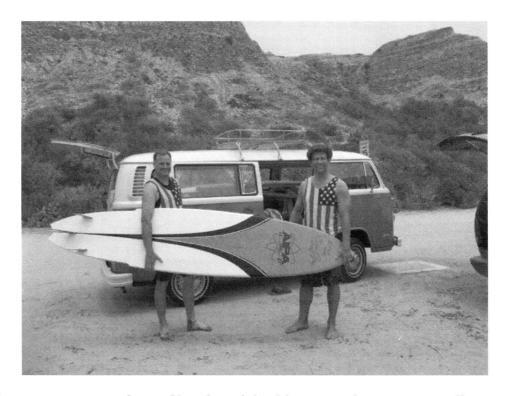

Johnny Z at San Onofre surf beach with buddy, Eric. Johnny is at 184 lbs. in year seven after his weight loss after initiating the Z-FAST method of maintaining a lifetime commitment weight. FASTING WORKS!

THE PROMISE

Once you determine your lifetime commitment weight, you need to make a sincere and wholehearted promise to reach and maintain that number. For example, if your goal is 180 pounds, you make a vow to yourself to never go above that weight, no matter what. It is an absolute maximum.

I recommend writing your vow down on a piece of paper.

Research shows that the action of writing and saying your goal out loud creates a better opportunity for success.

Write down on an index card or a piece of paper the following:

"I will never exceed (insert weight) lbs. again in my life. Ever. Under no circumstances will I go above (insert weight)."

Post this card in a place that you can view.

I keep mine near my scale.

When you go over your lifetime commitment weight (I usually go over mine 1–2 times per month) you will FAST for a full day. (More on this in the following chapter where Z–FAST is discussed in detail.)

If you Z–FAST, you will be amazed at how simple it will be to lose weight and maintain your lifetime commitment weight.

Okay, ready to learn about the different types of Z–FASTS?

CHAPTER ELEVEN

Z-FAST METHOD – LET'S GET STARTED!

"It's much easier to turn food off for one or two days a month than to try to portion and diet for the rest of your life on a daily basis."

— Johnny Z

Are you ready to discover the simplicity of Z-FASTING?

Ready to join the Z-FAST revolution?

Ready to get that beach body?

(Which means, of course, getting your body to the beach!)

There are THREE types of intermittent Z-FASTs:

❶ **The Systematic FAST** is used to drop weight (10–50 pounds).

❷ **The Scheduled FAST** (and the spontaneous fast) is used to maintain weight.

❸ **The Intervention FAST** is for when you've gone above your target weight and need an intervention STAT. (And yes, you will need it from time to time!)

3 Intermittent Fasting Methods: Z-FAST

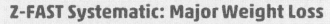

01

Z-FAST Systematic: Major Weight Loss
- 1/2-day fast 1 time per week
- Full Fast 1 time per week
- Normal eating outside fast days

02

Scheduled Z-FAST: Maintain Your Weight
- Weekly 1/2-day fast
- 1 full-day fast once a month
- Spontaneous fasting

03

Z-FAST Intervention: Lifetime Weight Commitment
- Immediate fast when over your commitment weight
- Keep your promise
- Weigh yourself daily

1. THE Z-FAST SYSTEMATIC METHOD

The Systematic Fast is useful for those looking to lose a significant amount of weight such as 10–50 pounds to reach a lifetime commitment weight as I did.

How it works:

This approach begins with two fasts a week for up to 50 weeks. One day is a HALF FAST and one day is a FULL FAST. Maintain this schedule until you reach your lifetime commitment weight. That's it!

For instance, you do a full fast every Wednesday (no breakfast, lunch, or dinner) and a half fast on Mondays (no breakfast and lunch). See chart below for the Full Fast Schedule. The half-day fast is easier where you only skip breakfast and lunch and have zero calories until dinner.

My Monthly Z-FAST: Systematic Weight Loss						
M	T	W	TH	F	S	S
M	T	W	TH	F	S	S
M	T	W	TH	F	S	S
M	T	W	TH	F	S	S

● 1/2-Day Fast ▦ Full-Day Fast

4 Full-Fast Days per Month
4 Half-Day Fasts per Month

Example of a Full Day Z-FAST on a Wednesday: skipping all meals, eating no food, taking in no calories, only water, and black coffee.

How to get started:

(It's super easy!)

1) Set a target weight that is manageable.

2) Make a chart or use the one provided here (also downloadable at www.ZFAST.us).

3) Chart your weight each morning.

4) Tell your spouse, kids, or friends about your goal.

5) Pick your best day to fast and tell others, "I'm fasting."

6) Ask for help and support. Research shows that soliciting help towards a goal will elicit long-term results.

7) Confirm at 7 a.m. the morning of your fast that no matter what, you are fasting. This means saying "no" even if you encounter:

- Free lunch and snacks
- Special cookies available
- Birthday cake
- Tempting "favorite" dinner
- Free pizza day
- Free candy
- A chocolate egg on your doorstep from the Easter Bunny

NO MATTER WHAT!

8) Fixate on your reward. Think about how great you will feel at 7 p.m. when you make it. What an accomplishment! You're a faster and you dropped fat right off your belly.

9) Do not tempt yourself with even one bite, one chip, one power bar, one sip of juice, etc. That, my friends, is what I called a slippery slope and you will slide.

10) You're eating NOTHING!

11) Absolutely NO CALORIES — even liquid calories. No juicing, power shakes, etc.

12) On the day that you are fasting, reduce all peer pressure to "have a little something" by announcing to others that you are fasting, especially if you are at lunch or dinner.

13) Drink caffeine to keep an edge and always hydrate (I chug 16 oz. sparkling water for lunch).

14) Get tons of hydration. Drink water or any hydrating liquids, but nothing with calories.

15) If you're feeling dizzy and think you can't make it, you're likely drinking too much caffeine (with no food to absorb it) and not enough water.

16) Push through the psychological aspect. Your body craves calories, but you DON'T NEED THEM. You have fat stores. Keep going, and you will enjoy all the benefits and results of a healthier body.

17) Think about those who have succeeded at fasting. (Jesus and Moses each went 40 days! Gandhi went 21 days with only sips of water!)

18) You can give up the pain (dedicate the fast) to someone else, a higher cause, and think about that person and cause throughout the day. Don't let them down by eating.

19) At dinner, you can sit down with family and friends (what I do) or skip the social event altogether if it is too tempting.

20) The Z-FAST provides the opportunity to reward yourself after 7 p.m. if you choose. If you'd like to think about this during the day, it may help you make it through:

    - Go to bed early (ahhh ... no housework).
    - Enjoy a straight vodka martini, wine, or juice under 100 calories. (These are my favorite rewards.)
    - Read the book you've wanted to read, binge watch that TV series, or work on your hobby.

21) After 8:30 p.m. be ready for the best sleep of the month. With no food to keep the body digesting and working all night, you will fall asleep like a baby.

You'll sleep all night and likely have trouble getting up in the morning, even after eight solid hours.

Finally, wake up and celebrate!

You made it through a 32-hour FAST.

Have breakfast or skip food until lunch like I usually do and keep the calories out and fat-burning happening even longer.

On the following page you'll find a monthly glance at a systematic weight loss method, where you commit to the whole month of the weekly Z-FAST method. You will drop weight like never before.

Z-FAST Systematic Weight Loss

MON	TUES	WED	THUR	FRI	SAT	SUN
B	B	X	B	B	B	B
L	L	X	L	L	L	L
D	D	X	D	D	D	D
B	B	X	B	B	B	B
L	L	X	L	L	L	L
D	D	X	D	D	D	D
B	B	X	B	B	B	B
L	L	X	L	L	L	L
D	D	X	D	D	D	D
B	B	X	B	B	B	B
L	L	X	L	L	L	L
D	D	X	D	D	D	D

1 Full Fast + 1 Half-Day Fast Once a Week
6-12 Weeks

Weigh in every day. Watch your weight drop by fasting.

Download the following chart on the www.ZFAST.us website.

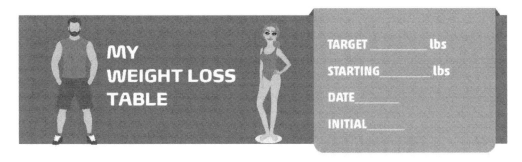

My Systematic Weight Loss Plan: Z-FAST

Date	Weight	Fast

My goal is to lose _____ lbs
in _____ weeks by Z-FAST methods

My Typical "Next Days" After Fasting

I skip breakfast the next day.

My stomach is smaller due to going one day without food (yes, it happens that quickly!), so I usually eat less at lunch.

I am so thankful for food; I make healthier choices when choosing my post-fast meal.

A benefit at dinner is now my stomach is still shrunken, and there's NO way I can eat a big meal.

Excellent!

I feel full and eat less than usual.

WOOHOO!

After the fast, I'm back under my lifetime commitment weight of 185.0 pounds. REMEMBER THE DECIMAL!

Now it's time to party on the weekend!

When Saturday rolls around, I eat what I want with no worries.

Now I can be loose with the family and friends and have fun without fretting over counting calories or weight gain.

I surf on Saturday, which is my routine exercise.

On Sunday I enjoy a tasty brunch with eggs, sausage, and toast followed with a fantastic evening rib-eye BBQ including the red wine.

I walk AND surf on Sunday, so I do NOT skip the rib-eye!

Since I did so well with my fast on Wednesday and endured the pain, there is no way I am skipping my favorite meal.

On Monday I weigh myself, and I'm at 184.1.

I am below my target weight goal, so all is good for the week.

Fasting — see you in a couple of weeks!

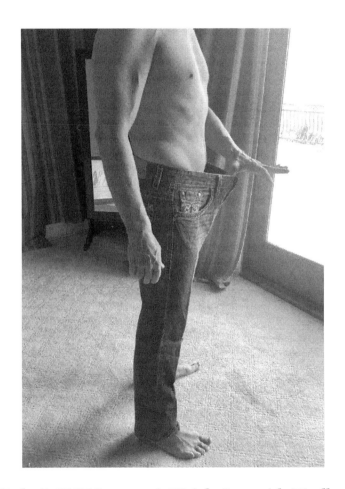

AFTER the Z-FAST Systematic Weight Loss with 20+ lbs. gone.

No more "over forty" man belly.

Join the Z-FAST revolution!

The Evening Reward

When I complete an entire day of fasting, I will reward myself with a beverage, usually a vodka martini which has zero carbs and very few calories, a small glass of wine, or an occasional beer.

If alcohol is not your thing, then allow yourself the reward of a little 4–6 ounces of apple juice or some other fruit juice.

The key is to pick a beverage reward that will not exceed 100 calories.

I believe it's essential that your reward be liquid rather than a cookie, cracker, or something solid. It's just too easy to continue eating once you start. Better to stick with the liquid reward and no more.

I find that having an alcoholic beverage after fasting improves my mood significantly and enables me to fall asleep very quickly that night. You can pick a different reward such as just going to bed early and skipping the housework.

Nighty-Night!

Speaking of sleep, I always sleep better on fast days than on any other day.

First, there are no digestive operations are happening to interrupt my sleep: no upset stomach, or a too-full tummy when hitting the pillow.

Two, cravings usually last 20–30 minutes after lunch and dinner (for me it's chocolate). But since I've fasted all day, these cravings don't interfere with my sleep.

Three, I find that my body is so ready for sleep after a fasting day that I have trouble getting up the next morning after my restful night. I could comfortably sleep an extra hour. When there are no calories added to my body for the day, it's easier for my body to shut down for sleep.

Four, there is no glucose flowing in my stomach to keep me wired and awake.

That's why I suggest that you reward yourself with an early nighttime retirement on your fasting day and enjoy a deep and restful night's sleep.

What to Expect When Beginning Your Z-FAST Intermittent Fasting Lifestyle

I want to be upfront and honest with you.

Unless you're a seasoned faster, the first few times you fast for an entire 24–30 hours, it is going to be an adjustment.

I promise you that after you master those first few days, fasting gets easier every time.

Your body becomes accustomed to handling a fast.

But I feel it's important that you're aware of what to expect when you start your Z-FAST lifestyle, so you're not caught off guard and feel like giving up!

Everyone is different, and so everyone has a different experience.

The first few times I fasted, my body was screaming for calories and glucose. My stomach rumbled loudly, and I experienced headaches. Some of those headaches were mild but, on a few occasions, they were worse than others.

(If a headache persists or is too intense, I will take ibuprofen on a rare occasion.)

You can reduce or eliminate headaches by staying hydrated!

Having a cup of black coffee around 3 p.m. also helps relieve headaches.

If you can make it past your first full day of fasting, you are 90% likely to make it happen the second, third, and fourth time and lose that weight for a lifetime!

Each time you fast, it gets easier and easier. Your confidence will grow!

For example, I no longer experience those headaches that I had at the outset of my commitment to make the Z-FAST a lifestyle choice.

A Note on Coffee

Coffee is an essential part of my fasting days, so I'm very thankful for the newer studies that show it benefits health and can help with weight loss and fasting success.

It also assists with fat-burn: studies show that caffeine can increase the burning of fat by as much as 10% in the obese and 29% for others.[15] How great is this?!

Caffeine is found in nearly all commercial fat-burning supplement. It's one of the very few natural substances that has been shown to aid fat-burning. Several studies even show that caffeine can boost the metabolic rate by 3–11%.[16] So, for all you coffee drinkers out there, HURRAY!

Aside from burning fat, coffee has been shown to fight depression.

In a 2011 Harvard study, it was proven that women who consumed four or more cups of coffee per day had a 20% lower risk of becoming depressed.[17]

Donald Hensrud, M.D. of the Mayo Clinic, said, "Studies have shown that coffee may have health benefits, including protecting against Parkinson's disease, Type 2 diabetes, liver disease, and liver cancer. Coffee also appears to improve cognitive function and decrease the risk of depression."[18]

---

[15] www.healthline.com/nutrition/coffee-increase-metabolism#section3

[16,17,18] Hensrud M.D., Donald. "The Surprising Health Benefits of Coffee." Mayo Clinic, Mayo Foundation for Medical Education and Research, 4 Mar. 2017, www.mayoclinic.org/healthy-lifestyle/nutrition-and-healthy-eating/expert-answers/coffee-and-health/faq-20058339

Coffee has been shown to increase metabolism, and even improve libido in some women.

Go, Girls, Go!

Body Cravings Are Evidence of Fat-Burning

The afternoon cravings happen when your body asks for sugar and glucose to go into the bloodstream. Your body is so used to having sugar and calories constantly shoveled in throughout the day that it goes into shock: "Hey, where's the food you're always feeding me?"

The cravings kick in. Your body cries out for the calories it's accustomed to.

FEED ME! FEED ME!

When you master those moments and choose to have a cup of black coffee or a delicious sparkling water instead of giving in, YOU WIN BIG.

When you don't eat, your body will automatically get energy from fat stores.

You just have to make it through that short period of 1–2 hours, and you'll be home free.

Remind yourself to equate the slight discomfort and craving pain as proof that the weight loss and fat-burning wheels are turning!

Ignore those cravings because you know you're burning fat. This is the increased metabolic rate happening.

Feel proud of those moments when you win, and where you make it!

You'll feel the loss of almost one pound of fat over the FAST period.

Yes, one pound!

Your body will be working differently.

There's that tingling as the fat-burning machine kicks in.

YES! YES!

(I'll have what she's having!)

See yourself in that old pair of your favorite jeans from college.

Imagine how you'll look in that swimsuit you've had your eye on.

All you have to do is NOT eat, and you'll feel your body jump-starting the fat-burning process and dropping pounds.

Those cravings will come to be recognized as pure joy!

The Post-Fast Day

After a full day of fasting for 24–30 hours, you'll find that your stomach has shrunk significantly. You'll eat less the day afterward, plus you won't want to undo the weight loss you earned from your previous day of fasting.

You'll only be hungry for 1/2 a sandwich when you usually eat an entire one, or you'll skip the chips or fries that you ordinarily would have ordered along with the big sandwich.

You won't be as hungry because your stomach has shrunk. Believe me when I tell you that greasy food just WILL NOT appeal to you.

Most people think that after a day of fasting you'll go crazy and stuff your face with food. It's exactly the opposite.

Your body will crave clean, healthier foods, which will taste delicious for sure!

You can't imagine how much you'll enjoy food when you've gone without.

> **"When you don't have food in your life, just for a day, it makes you realize you're lucky to have it the next day. So, the day after fasting, the music that comes out will be very joyous."**
>
> — Chris Martin, Coldplay

By the time dinner rolls around, your stomach will be smaller than before your fast day, so you will eat less than you ordinarily would have eaten.

It's kind of like being in the desert and having no water for an extended period. When you finally have access to water, if you drink too much of it too fast, you throw it up because your body cannot handle too much of it.

It's the same with food on the day after a fast. You won't want to overindulge. If you do, you won't feel well.

By the end of the post-fast day, you will undoubtedly lose some additional weight because you will not have consumed a full 2,500–3,000 calories that day.

You may have only consumed 50% of that. It's the second-day weight loss bonus!

The Recap

You've lost a pound after a complete 24–30 hour fast. You've burned hardcore fat. Your stomach shrank, which resulted in your consuming fewer calories the day following your fast.

The net result of one complete day of fasting could add up to up to a two-pound weight loss including your post-fast day.

BAM! You are back to your lifetime commitment weight.

Additionally, you slept like a baby. Plus, your human growth hormones increased 2,000% if you're a male and 1,300% if you're a female, your insulin levels decreased, your metabolism increased, and you now control the power over food.

By the time the weekend rolls around, you'll be back to eating your 2,500–3,000 calories.

However, you'll realize that you don't need that extra slice of pizza or handful of chips when you aren't starving.

You have already proven through your fasting that you hold power over food, not vice versa.

The fast gives you the power over the weekends to say no to some of the extras calories.

And so, the positive fasting cycle begins!

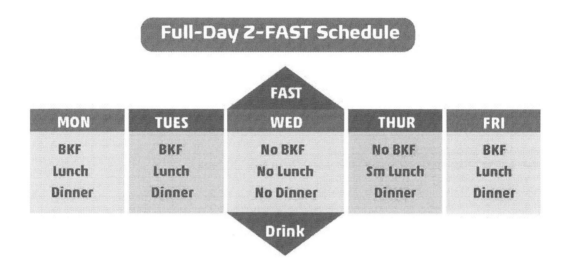

2. THE Z-FAST SCHEDULED FAST:
MAINTAIN YOUR WEIGHT

Congratulations! You've lost weight by utilizing the Z-FAST Systematic Method by using weekly full and half-day fasts!

You have reached the weight on your scale you haven't seen in years!

You've received a lot of compliments, too.

You've dedicated and disciplined yourself, followed instructions, and achieved your lifetime commitment weight. But you've probably been here before after losing weight, just like millions of other Americans.

It's seems losing the weight is the easiest part. Keeping it off is the challenge.

The SCHEDULED FAST is useful for individuals looking to maintain their lifetime commitment weight.

How it works:

This approach follows a monthly schedule.

One FULL-DAY FAST per month.

Three HALF-DAY FASTS per month (breakfast and lunch skipped).

My Monthly Z-FAST: Maintain						
M	T	W	TH	F	S	S
M	T	W	TH	F	S	S
M	T	W	TH	F	S	S
M	T	W	TH	F	S	S

●1/2-Day Fast ■Full-Day Fast

1 Full-Day Fast Per Month: NO breakfast, NO lunch, NO dinner
3 Half-Day Fasts Per Month: NO breakfast, NO lunch

So how does this work to maintain a LIFETIME COMMITMENT WEIGHT?

Remember that the National Institute of Health reported that most dieters fail to keep off the weight they lose, and most gain back MORE THAN THEY LOST. Their conclusion was, "there is little support for the notion that diets lead to lasting weight loss or health benefits."

It may be easy to go on a weight loss program for a short period until you lose a few, or maybe even a lot of pounds. But to be truly successful, the change has to be a commitment to **staying on a program for life**.

That's where all these other diets fail. They're too hard to maintain indefinitely.

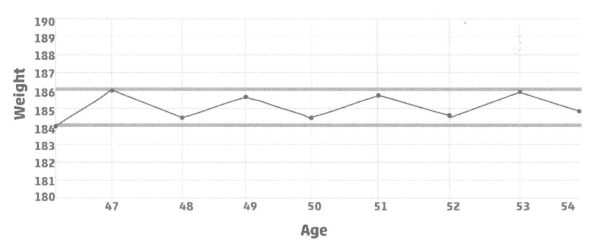

Lifetime Weight Commitment

Never Exceed Maximum Limit Without
An Interventional Z-FAST

7-Year History Using Z-FAST Method — Keeping
My Lifetime Weight Commitment

How can you possibly stay on the Atkins diet for life?

How can you maintain a way of eating where you must portion food every day for every single meal for the rest your life?

It just won't happen.

You're set up to fail.

In comparison to the other diets, it's pretty darn easy to take a few days a month **to close the door on calories.** If you can do that, you can live a healthy life while eating the food and beverages you love (with reasonable moderation of course).

Z-FAST is a lifelong program to ensure you maintain that success. This is where the Scheduled and Interventional fasts come into play as a component of your commitment to never go beyond your lifetime goal weight again.

Share your good news!

I have advised many people that you are not on a "diet" until you have told other people that:

❶ You are on a diet; and

❷ You have a lifetime commitment weight to uphold.

If you have already achieved your weight goal, let your spouse, family, friends, and co-workers know that as part of your commitment to your lifetime weight, that you will need an intermittent fast from time to time to maintain it and this will now be your new lifestyle.

Explain to those people that you worked hard to achieve your lifetime commitment weight (hand them my book), tell that you feel great and that you will be maintaining this schedule for the rest of your life. They will understand when you have to pass on a lunch invitation, drinks after work, a slice of party cake, etc. They will admire you for your dedication. They won't take it personally when you ask for a "rain check" on happy hour, and they may even be a little envious of your ability to resist caloric temptations (as well as how doggone great you look).

A word of advice: be sure to let your spouse or partner know when it's a fasting day, so they don't unknowingly make a big dinner and expect you to eat it with them. (I learned the hard way and had an upset wife on several occasions.)

I was born in the Midwest and was raised on meat and potatoes. I now reside in California where everyone is (as is commonly known) a "little crazy" about health. Discussing the Z-FAST in California is no big deal in the land where everyone is striving to look their best.

Maybe in your neck of the woods, it's a little different, and fasting would be considered out of the ordinary. In such an environment, it's even more critical that you explain the reasons why you have committed to intermittent fasting, and perhaps explain the scientific benefits behind it. You might gather a few recruits!

A Note About the Office/Work

Let's talk about the workplace or your job.

When I'm fasting, I let my co-workers know that it's a fasting day for me.

(After a while, people noticed when I wasn't taking lunch and would ask, "Is it a fasting day, John?")

I've found that my co-workers are very supportive and interested in this lifestyle of intermittent fasting that I've committed to. They congratulate me on my discipline. The reality is that I'm probably putting in less work at losing weight than they are, and I'm winning the battle.

Some say they can't understand how I can go without food for an entire day until I explain the Z-FAST to them.

Others have joined me in committing to this lifestyle choice — and have encouraged me to write this book about how and when to go on an intermittent fast successfully.

Still other co-workers reveal that they too fast for religious reasons at different times of the year and understand my commitment to my Z-FAST lifestyle choice. (See Chapter Nine for more on religious fasting.)

If you are open and uninhibited about your commitment to intermittent fasting with your co-workers, it will make it that much easier to resist the caloric temptations on a fasting day. Plus, you will undoubtedly receive encouragement and gain supporters for your dedication like I do.

Weigh In Every Day for the Moment of Truth

I know this sounds crazy, but if you have been monitoring your weight every day and you step on the scale and the moment of truth meets your eye — you'll have a much easier time maintaining your weight.

By monitoring your weight daily, you'll never again allow that creeping weight gain to happen to you. This is a special secret of the Z-FAST.

You'll have a lifetime commitment to your ideal weight and health WITHOUT using any fancy diets or extreme exercise regimens.

That's why I recommend keeping a chart of your daily weight. Keep it close to your scale along with a pen or record it on your mobile phone where it won't get lost (and can travel with you). It takes a minute to jump on the scale and record your weight. After a while, this activity will be automatic and be part of your regular daily routine. It will seriously help you drop and maintain weight!

When I'm on vacation, I don't always have the opportunity (or desire) to fast, but I will certainly fast and drop an extra pound before I leave, and sometimes order a scale from housekeeping, if possible.

3. THE Z-FAST INTERVENTIONAL FAST:
NEVER GAIN WEIGHT AGAIN

This "when-needed fast" is critical to keeping your lifetime commitment weight!

Since you weigh yourself daily, if you find that you're over your lifetime commitment weight for two consecutive days, then you must do a Z-FAST Intervention IMMEDIATELY.

This is straightforward to do, and I do it myself when this happens to me. (And this does happen to me.)

If by chance you have a business dinner or a significant commitment involving a meal (like your wedding), then fast a day later but DO NOT delay any longer than that. No extensions and no excuses! Don't wait until the weekend; it will be too late.

The Interventional Fast is used in addition to any regular half-day scheduled fasts, and it will immediately cure a weight gain.

Since you weigh yourself daily, if you find that you are over your lifetime commitment weight for two consecutive days, do a Z-FAST Intervention IMMEDIATELY.

How it works:

At this point, you've achieved your lifetime commitment weight after using the Systematic Fast.

The first step begins with a self-discovery process to determine what weight on the scale makes you happiest and healthiest.

What number do you not want to go above?

(Remember that decimal!)

This is your number, not your friend's number, the government's recommended number, or any other number.

It is YOUR number that makes you whole, and it has to be realistic and manageable.

Don't start with your high school wrestling weight or your high school prom dress weight just yet.

FYI the decimal HAS to be used.

In my case, it's 185.0.

Not 185.6 or 185.3

Without a decimal, it doesn't work.

See this chart for reference on what can happen without the decimal:

Weight	Date	Comment
185.1	Oct	great
185.4	Oct	it's nothing big
184.9	Oct	I'm fine
185.9	Oct	just noise
186.3	Nov	hmmm
186.2	Nov	going down
186.7	Nov	still there
186.6	Nov	See, going down
186.9	Nov	but not down, need help
187.5	Nov	shit, I'm way over

I had to learn the hard way (see above, because that is WITHOUT FASTING).

These days, my target weight goal is hardcore with a decimal: 185.0 and not a fraction higher.

Lifetime Weight Management Through Fasting

When to Intervene

#	Calories	Day	Status
Day 1	183.9	FRI	OK
Day 2	185.1	SAT	OK
Day 3	184.6	SUN	OK
Day 4	185.4	MON	OVER
Day 5	186.5	TUE	OVER
Day 6	Fast	WED	FAST INTERVENTION
Day 7	184.6	THUR	OK
Day 8	184.3	FRI	OK
Day 9	183.2	SAT	OK
Day 10	184.0	SUN	OK

If you are over your lifetime commitment weight 2 days in a row, you will fast starting within 24 hours
No Exceptions!

I will never weigh 185-something (at least not for more than one or two days).

A few rules:

There will be fluctuation, but it must be *under* your goal, not over.

If your weight is over your target goal for two days in a row, it's an automatic fast the following day.

That second-day weigh-in decides if an immediate fast is necessary.

When you go over your number, you will be fasting the next day.

PERIOD.

The Lifetime Weight of 185.0 is breached two days in a row. I don't start the Atkins diet, daily portioning, or an intense exercise routine. I simply don't eat for ONE day. I Z-FAST, drop the weight, and go back to my normal life. DONE. Of course, I'll be a little more careful. But it's that easy. EIGHT years at 185.0 is the proof!

Days 4 and 5 in the chart shows that my weight went up and over the target two days in a row. Time to FAST!

I could wait to reach 187 before I fast, but I guarantee I'll be flirting with even more weight gain if I do.

I tailor my intermittent fast depending on how much I have exceeded my commitment weight.

For instance, if I haven't exceeded my commitment weight by too much, I may decide to first fast one or two days by skipping breakfast and lunch and eating only dinner only (and NO gorging). If I'm still not at 185.0 or lower when I weigh myself the morning,

I'll do a full day fast for 24–30 hours. I will not eat any food, but I will drink black coffee, water, and zero-calorie liquids throughout the day.

(Personally, I load up on sparkling water as it's very filling).

I feel empowered when I'm able to fast and stop eating food altogether. I have power over food because I know how to fast.

Try it and see.

Make your commitment to never go over your lifetime weight goal!

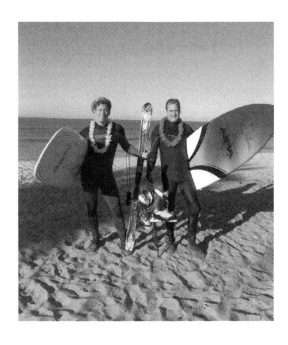

California "Combo Day: surf and snow ski on the same day at 184 lbs. after doing an Interventional Fast the week before to keep my weight in check to be downhill ready!

When to Intervene: Z-FAST Example

Do Not Stay Over Target More Than 24 Hours: Make the Promise

MON	TUES	WED	THUR	FRI	SAT	SUN
184 lbs	183 lbs	185 lbs	184 lbs	183 lbs	183 lbs	182 lbs
B	B	B	B	B	B	B
L	L	L	L	L	L	L
D	D	D	D	D	D	D
183 lbs	182 lbs	182 lbs	182 lbs	184 lbs	184.5 lbs	185.0 lbs
B	B	B	B	B	B	B
L	L	L	L	L	L	L
D	D	D	D	D	D	D
186 lbs	186 lbs	Z-FAST INTERVENE	183 lbs	184 lbs	184 lbs	184 lbs
B	B	B̶	B	B	B	B
L	L	X	L	L	L	L
D	D	D̶	D	D	D	D
184 lbs 1/2-Day Fast	183 lbs	183 lbs	184 lbs	185 lbs	184 lbs	185 lbs
B̶	B	B	B	B	B	B
X	L	L	L	L	L	L
D	D	D	D	D	D	D

Everybody likes a little spontaneity, right?

This brings me to the **Spontaneous Fast**. You'll employ this fast when it's convenient, such as when there's an opportunity to skip a meal due to extenuating circumstances such as:

- Dropping off kids
- Running late for lunch
- Too busy to eat
- Traveling

- Having to eat in a rush

- Working and too late for a lunchtime meal

- Flying, or

- Any instance where meals are interrupted

Skip it and count it as a fasting day!

Put that time you would have dedicated to eating back into your life.

Hello, extra time!

Hello, fat burn!

Hello, smarty-pants!

If you're on the move, you've run out of time, or if you didn't find something to eat that you wanted, or that project is due, then skip the meal and FAST.

Everybody loves a freebie!

When spontaneously fasting, this skipped meal can count as a fast day and can replace one of your scheduled fasting days.

You don't have to plan and think about the fast, but still be able to skip a meal, reduce calorie intake, burn fat, get ready for the weekend, and get all the other benefits of a healthy fasting day.

I skip breakfast daily to gain as much fasting time as possible and gain some fat-burning time before lunch. So, when I'm able to pass on a meal, I get a great day of fasting and burning fat: a half-day freebie.

I love this opportunity, and regularly take advantage of it and urge you to do so too!

You get the full benefit of fasting from lunch one day until lunch the next day (24 hours) by skipping dinner and not eating until breakfast the next day (18 hours).

I fast spontaneously about 30% of the time to make sure I complete my scheduled maintenance fasts during the month and lower my interventional emergency fasts.

For instance, I have a scheduled half-fast on my usual Monday. Say I'm super busy at work during lunch on Thursday (which is a non-planned day to fast) and yet it was effortless to skip lunch due to running late so I do so.

I will then have one extra fast "in the bank" so to speak and can decide whether I want to take this as an extra or replace it with my schedule Wednesday fast.

This also limits the number of INTERVENTION FASTS I need to complete.

This can also work for dinner.

You and I are likely not accustomed to skipping dinner, and except for fasting, I never miss it.

(Well, maybe once in college.)

But if the chance arises, and since you are now conscious of the health benefits of FASTING, and you could quietly and effortlessly skip dinner, as they say: JUST DO IT.

Z-FAST Schedule to Maintain Health / Weight

	MON	TUES	WED	THUR	FRI	SAT	SUN
1/2-Day Fast	B̶	B	B	B	B	B	B
	L̶	L	L	L	L	L	L
	D	D	D	D	D	D	D
1/2-Day Fast				**Spontaneous Fast**			
	B̶	B	B	B̶	B	B	B
	L̶	L	L	L̶	L	L	L
	D	D	D	D	D	D	D
1/2-Day Fast							
	B̶	B	B	B	B	B	B
	L̶	L	L	L	L	L	L
	D	D	D	D	D	D	D
			Full Fast				
	B	B	B̶	B	B	B	B
	L	L	L̶	L	L	L	L
	D	D	D̶	D	D	D	D

A tip to skipping dinner is to have another activity available from your to-do list where you can quickly replace the habit of eating. A dinner skip is fantastic, especially when you go without breakfast the morning following.

Slam the door on weight gain: ONE DAY AND DONE!

I have maintained my commitment weight for EIGHT YEARS because I made the promise to myself that I would never go above 185.0.

I have weighed 185.0 or less 99.9% of the time because WHEN I do go over (and it CAN and WILL happen from time to time), I immediately and unconditionally go on a FULL ONE DAY INTERVENTION FAST.

You too must do the same.

Repeat after me, "I will NEVER, EVER, EVER for any reason, no matter what, exceed my lifetime commitment weight without immediate fasting intervention."

I suggest you tell your spouse, family, friends, and coworkers about the lifetime commitment you have made never to exceed your ideal weight goal of _____ lbs. (fill in your target weight).

By vocalizing your intentions and making it known, you increase your likelihood of succeeding in maintaining your lifelong weight commitment. You worked hard to achieve this ideal weight.

I enjoy the significant health benefits I feel during a fast, too!

No, I'm not a masochist, but it feels good to know I have the power to control my health.

The scientific evidence for the benefits of intermittent fasting is substantial, as you saw in Chapter Seven. I enjoy knowing my human growth hormone increases, my insulin levels drop dramatically, and my acuity sharpens. Heck, I can feel it!

Advantages of Intermittent Fasting

One-Day Fasting Advantages

1) You'll dedicate one day vs. months of rigid diet commitment.

2) Your body systems will attack fat stores for energy.

3) You'll eat and drink as usual except on the day of the fast.

4) You'll get some great sleep.

5) You'll jumpstart your metabolism to burn fat and boost Human Growth Hormone to build muscle.

6) You'll experience that shrunken stomach bonus for two days more.

7) You'll say "no" to extras — which stop an extra FAST day!

Long-Term Fasting Advantages

1) You'll access new system for energy: stored FAT.

2) You'll clean out your GI tract.

3) You'll develop discipline over continuous feeding and the overabundance of food.

4) Your Human Growth Hormone will increase to build muscle.

5) You'll experience a hydration flush.

6) Your insulin levels will improve dramatically.

7) You'll increase your longevity.

8) You'll have a metabolism booster to burn fat.

9) You'll experience potential cancer-fighting benefits.

Remember to keep your lifetime commitment weight chart near your scale to record your daily weigh-ins. This quick and easy daily routine will keep you on track and alert you to when an Interventional Fast is necessary.

Lifetime Weight Commitment

_____ lbs

INTERVENE WITH Z-FAST

Date	Weight	Fast

I will never exceed more than _____ lbs in my life

without 24-hour intervention through fasting!

Here are all my interventions for the year 2016. Not too bad. I kept all the weight off and lived a fun, happy life. I ate what I wanted on ALL the other days.

My 52-WEEK CHART FOR 1 YEAR Z-FAST INTERVENTIONS 2016

AVERAGE WEEKLY WEIGHT AND FASTS

Maintain a tight range on the upper limits.
Immediate FAST and intervention when exceeding lifetime weight commitment. Looking at the big picture, it is easy! Only 8 full-day fasts & 2 half-day fasts!

MANAGE YOUR WEIGHT

week				week			
week	1	183.5	FAST	week	27	186.2	FAST
week	2	183.6		week	28	186.4	
week	3	183.7		week	29	185.4	
week	4	183.8		week	30	184.4	
week	5	183.9		week	31	183.9	
week	6	184.0	FAST	week	32	184.5	
week	7	184.1		week	33	185.2	
week	8	184.2		week	34	185.3	1/2-Day Fast
week	9	184.3		week	35	184.8	
week	10	184.1	Full FAST	week	36	184.9	
week	11	184.5		week	37	184.7	
week	12	186.2		week	38	184.1	
week	13	186.4		week	39	184.3	
week	14	185.4		week	40	184.1	
week	15	184.4		week	41	183.9	
week	16	183.9		week	42	185.0	FAST
week	17	184.5	1/2-Day Fast	week	43	183.9	
week	18	185.2		week	44	183.3	
week	19	185.3		week	45	183.1	
week	20	184.8		week	46	184.3	
week	21	184.9		week	47	182.7	
week	22	184.7		week	48	182.5	
week	23	184.1	FAST	week	49	183.7	FAST
week	24	184.3		week	50	182.9	
week	25	184.1		week	51	183.1	
week	26	183.9		week	52	185.0	
				week	1	186.0	FAST

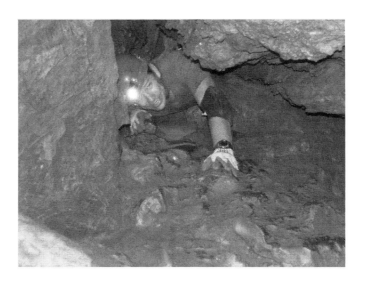

Fitting through "Pancake Alley" during underground caving adventure after a Z-FAST one-time Interventional Full Fast, plus a half-day fast to burn off four lbs.

After dropping four lbs., I was able to squeeze my way through underground caves like a pro!

CHAPTER TWELVE

Fasting Success Stories

DR. WILLIAM F. NORTHRUP III, MD

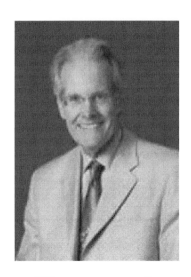

Edina, Minnesota

Cardiac Surgeon, Corporate VP

"Fasting makes more sense for weight loss than exercise. I use a full fast to maintain my life commitment weight."

William F. Northrup III, MD is Vice President of Physician Relations and Education at CryoLife and a heart surgeon. He spent nearly three decades in clinical practice in the Twin Cities of Minneapolis and St. Paul, Minnesota, primarily focused on heart surgery.

This is his testimony:

Fasting makes more sense for weight loss than exercise.

I use a full fast to maintain my life commitment weight. I have been skipping breakfast and lunch for many years and believe in a full 24 hour fast as a true fast.

I have a weight goal that I have been maintaining for many years of 155 lbs. I believe that eating fewer meals is the key.

I usually skip breakfast and lunch, and occasionally eat a handful of olives. I purposely stay busy, and I don't notice any energy level change when skipping meals.

As I age, I may have less energy, but it's not related to fasting.

I also look to decrease portions.

I don't take seconds.

I don't bring food home from restaurants ever as it means I ordered too much food.

Fasting closes the door on calories and thinking of food. It allows you to redirect your thoughts and use your time for something else. You can redirect energy and discipline to other things.

Not thinking about food enables you to spend time out making your marriage better, improving at work, delivering on other projects, spending time with kids, etc. You can spend a whole day thinking about food — like French-style creamy scrambled eggs — and with fasting, that discipline ends it.

Exercise alone won't do it. Walking a mile burns about 100 calories. It's like spitting in the wind for weight loss and is an ineffective way to lose weight. I work out on a treadmill with an annual goal of 365 hours/year but not for weight management, but for health reasons.

FASTING and eating less is what works for weight management.

Five Small Meals A Day: I don't buy it.

I looked at the study promoting five small meals a day, as that's what I do as a scientist, and the study is not that good or conclusive, and I don't buy it. I can lose three pounds in a week with fasting alone. I appreciate not having to constantly figure out portion control, as that doesn't work for me either. Five meals a day is not controllable.

A tip for fasting:

I gave up sugary drinks and desserts years ago, but in rare instances, I will have a soda. But I switched to soda stream. I love fizzy sparkling water and will have 1–2 glasses, which fill me up, especially versus regular water. The fizz and bubbles are great to help with meal skipping.

One thing I did was to set a goal to keep a specific weight and fast to stay there.

When you're fasting, you learn to appreciate healthier foods, too. For example, I'm all about salads now. I make my own vinaigrette. I love ceviche! Tuna, protein, olives, avocados — there are so many tasty foods.

I have committed to a lifetime weight and have kept it in check for 20 years.

I intermittently FAST at least two days a week. I skip breakfast and lunch. I rarely eat breakfast, no matter what.

I'm a cardiac heart surgeon and work in the corporate world now, so I certainly want to be on my game, and I know the benefits of a healthy lifestyle especially as it pertains to cardiovascular health.

FASTING has always been a good strategy for me. **It's so obvious, to not gain weight: DON'T EAT.**

— Dr. William F. Northrup III, MD, Edina Minnesota

JON RUBY

Lake Forest, CA
Professional Driver

I never saw a french fry I didn't like. And portioning was not happening. Calorie restriction was way too easy to cheat, as I always said that I would "start tomorrow.

But fasting works. I used it extensively as a secret to stay lean and maintain my desired weight.

My plan is to fast for an entire day, and by the end of the day, I always feel much better.

I feel a faster's high much like when I hit that six-mile marker of running.

I get this colossal endorphin rush when I fast, and this tingling in my stomach, just like a runner's high.

When I fast, I can feel something happening. I can feel the change as fat starts burning versus the feeling of burning the available food in my stomach.

In one day when you burn enough fat equaling the size or weight of a baked potato: you can feel that happening!

My advice is not to give up until the body provides the energy.

As a professional limousine driver, I have to be awake and aware during the day. My career depends on it!

You would think that I would be lethargic at the end of the day without eating, but once I start burning fat, I feel the real energy kick in. I use caffeine to stave off hunger and feel alert if I need to.

— Jon Ruby, Lake Forest, California

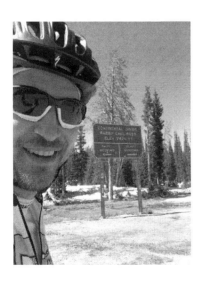

DAVE KING

Scottsdale, Arizona

Professional Sales Representative

DAVE KING fasts on Tuesdays, his best day to skip meals and maintain his lifetime commitment weight. Pictured here under his lifetime commitment weight of 175 lbs. Go Fasting!

I have committed to a lifetime weight and use fasting to maintain it.

I weigh in on Mondays. If I'm over, I fast the next day.

I choose Tuesday of every week to fast as it works well for me and my travel schedule. I'll fast one day, and by the end of the day I work out. I do not feel the energy drag.

The other significant advantage of fasting is that my stomach shrinks down big time. So, the next day or two I feel full on much smaller meals. That's one thing I love about fasting: that physical change in my stomach when nothing goes in it for 18–30 hours.

Also, fasting allows me to put time back on my schedule. Eating can use up a lot of time, especially when going out, so I save all that time and complete a project or work out (my favorite thing).

Here's my routine:

My target is 175 lbs. (a little more reasonable than my college weight). I prefer Monday and Tuesday for my weigh-in and fast days. I often do Tuesday away from home and find fasting is a little more comfortable if I'm not at home. I weigh myself Monday at the gym and allow a cushion of three lbs.

If I weigh in at 179 lbs, I begin my fast after dinner that same night.

I maintain a "Kitchen is Closed" policy after 8 p.m. no matter what, only drinking water before bed. The next day, I allow as much coffee and water as I can drink.

Tuesday evening, after the fast is over, I am always famished, but fill up quickly and usually eat less for dinner than I planned. This is an extra benefit of creating a small stomach: it's easier to become full.

I find the benefit of the fast always continues for a few days. My appetite does not come back with the same intensity I had before the fast. Since my stomach feels smaller, it also feels flatter.

Plus, I usually weigh 2–3 pounds lighter the following day, and I am faster on my bike.

I build momentum, so I work harder and eat healthier thanks to feeling lighter and more robust.

If I'm way over my target weight (maybe because of the holiday season), I have found that it never takes more than three or four fasting weeks to get back down to 175 pounds.

Now in my forties, I fast a few times a year — usually post-holidays, and after the Arizona summers — to cut weight for cycling events.

I've always believed in the benefits of putting an event on my calendar and training for it. Fasting and weekly monitoring of my weight until I hit my target provides the best kickstart for weight loss.

— Dave King, Scottsdale, Arizona

MICHAEL WILSON

Cape May, New Jersey

Owner/Head Strength & Conditioning Coach at Cape May Fitness & Sports

- **Certified Personal Trainer**
- **Certified USA Weightlifting Sports Performance Coach**
- **Certified Weightlifting Performance Coach – NSPA**

- **Certified Program Design – NSPA**
- **Certified Nutrition Coach – Precision Nutrition**

There is one method of exercise that has remained central to my training for the past 30 years ... resistance training!

I have implemented resistance training in various forms from bodybuilding and powerlifting to Olympic weightlifting and CrossFit, and I've had success using them all to get strong, fast and lean.

Despite my extensive experience implementing resistance training protocols, I admittedly lacked the proper nutritional knowledge necessary to maximize my results.

In my pursuit of knowledge, I enrolled in a comprehensive and rigorous 18-week nutrition certification course while simultaneously learning more about IF and how to implement it properly with exercise.

Except there was a small issue: all of the information I was reading regarding IF lacked practical, science-based advice on how to implement IF with resistance training. This left me frustrated, confused, and with more questions than answers.

I typically spend 16–20 hours in the fasted state with a feeding window of 4–8 hours, depending on which phase of IF I'm in. After two weeks of IF, I felt myself getting fuller much faster, which made sticking to my low-calorie diet quite manageable.

I know you're probably thinking, a low-calorie diet AND manageable, what's the catch? Well, luckily for us there really isn't one.

When you fast for extended periods of time your body begins to go through some pretty remarkable adaptations, most notably, your stomach begins to "shrink." Your stomach is a muscle that stretches and contracts just like your biceps stretch and contract during a bicep curl; and just like your biceps, the only time your stomach begins to "shrink" is when you stop stimulating it.

The latest science shows that fasting modifies the stomach on a cellular level and it begins to lose its willingness to stretch, thus making you feel fuller for longer.

Science has shown us that calorie intake is the driving force behind successfully losing weight, but dieting is so much more than calories in and calories out.

One of the biggest hurdles to overcome as a dieter, as many are aware, is the psychological aspect of having to eat less food and exercise more while simultaneously managing all of life's responsibilities.

As a coach, teacher, and business owner, IF gave me the ability to focus on my clients, students, and family while still achieving my body recomposition goals.

Put simply, IF allowed me to have my cake and eat it too!

At the start of my journey with IF I weighed a staggering 270 pounds. In less than two months I had dropped the easiest 28 pounds of my life without compromising my strength or mental sanity.

Fasting works!

— Mike Wilson, Cape May, New Jersey

CHAPTER THIRTEEN

Tips, Tricks & Summary

"If a man has nothing to eat, fasting is the most intelligent thing he can do."

— Hermann Hesse

You made it!

Congratulations on learning what Z-FAST is all about.

You ought to be feeling pretty good right about now!

... You've worked your way through the Z-FAST.

... You've educated yourself on all the benefits of intermittent fasting.

... You've read the testimonies of some folks who have used fasting on a long-term basis to lose weight, stay lean, feel sharp, and stay the heck off the Center for Disease Control's statistics list!

Ready to join the Z-FAST revolution?

We can't wait to have you join us!

Here's an example of my year:

ANNUAL FAST SCHEDULE: 2017 COMMITMENT
Maintain Weight — Z-FASTING ONLY

lbs

(M) 1/2-Day FAST= No Breakfast or Lunch
[W] Full-Day FAST= No Breakfast, Lunch or Dinner
☆ Interventional Full-Day

# of Full FASTS	1.2/Month	13 a Year
# of 1/2-Day FASTS	2/ Month	24 a Year
% of Z-FASTS that were Spontaneous		30%
% Time Spent Under 185.0 Target		95%+

As a recap ...

You know there are THREE types of fasting methods available to you:

❶ The Systematic FAST is a weekly fast used to drop weight (10–50 pounds).

❷ The Scheduled FAST (and the spontaneous fast) is used to maintain lost weight.

❸ The Intervention FAST is for when you've gone above your target weight and need an intervention STAT. (Blame it on my Midwest roots, but I can't help but be honest. You'll need it from time to time!)

You'll start by choosing your lifetime commitment weight.

You'll write down on an index card or a piece of paper the following: "I will never exceed XXX lbs. again in my life. Ever. Under no circumstances will I go above XXX number."

You'll post this card in a place that you can view often.

Using a combination of the Systematic, Scheduled, and Intervention fasts, you'll Z–FAST.

It's that easy.

Remember ...

Your body is ready to take advantage of all the benefits that intermittent fasting provides including:

- Better heart health (heart disease is the leading cause of death for Americans)

- Brain stimulant

- Cancer prevention and chemotherapy booster

- Increased autophagy (self-cannibalization, or cellular house-cleaning)

- Longer life (see above)

- Lower insulin (don't be a stat on developing Type 2 diabetes)

- Stimulate BHB (fight free radicals and inflammation)

- Stimulate Human Growth Hormone (feel sharper and stave off dementia-type disease)

- Stimulate that hungry stomach hormone, ghrelin (and develop more brain cells)

- Stimulate your metabolic rate (burn calories faster)

- Weight loss (eating fewer calories means weight loss)

- Not to mention ... you're going to look fabulous!

Here are a few tips and tricks to keep you on your feet, out of the kitchen, and smiling on the scale:

- Cravings are normal: stay busy or start a new task to work through it.

- Pick busy days to fast, so you're not concentrating on the eating routine.

- Don't be afraid of hunger: it's normal and will go away (remember that hunger stimulates the production of ghrelin, that cool little hormone that makes you smarter).

- Cravings last 20–30 minutes: drink sparkling water to fill your stomach until they pass.

- Water is your friend, drink as much as you can. (Help your cells clean house and flush toxins).

- Utilize caffeine. Drink black coffee or tea for a boost and pick-me-up.

- The first fast is the hardest and gets easier by far on #2 and #3. So, don't give in!

- Always get medical advice on weight loss and nutrition before beginning any routine.

So, what are you waiting for?

Now you're ready to change your life with my intermittent fasting system ...

Ready?

Set!

Z-FAST!

ABOUT THE AUTHOR

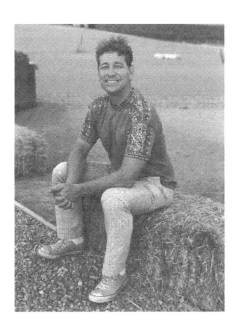

After experiencing that "post–40" creeping weight gain of 20+ pounds, John designed a personal fasting method that allowed him to lose that weight and keep it off for nearly a decade. After being repeatedly asked by friends, family members, and colleagues, "How do you stay so fit?" John Zehren (aka Johnny Z) decided it was time to tell the world about his fasting methods and start a new revolution with his book *Z-FAST: A Simple, Proven Intermittent Fasting Method* to lose weight for life. In Z-FAST, John shares his no-fail techniques for maintaining excellent physical and mental health and his proven program for losing that unwanted weight for life.

John tried all those popular diets, eating plans, and exercise regimens and expensive equipment purchases, but nothing worked for him. He needed quick and easy weight loss relief and a way of eating that matched his busy lifestyle. Balancing a family, career, and a full social life didn't allow for portioning, calorie and carb counting, extra gym time, or chasing down specialized food products. After vowing not to eat another bite of food until he was below 200 pounds, John discovered the ease and impressive results of intermittent fasting. Using the very methods described in this book, John easily lost 20 pounds. He can now testify to maintaining his ideal weight for over EIGHT YEARS STRAIGHT with zero yo-yo diet maintenance through Z-FAST methods.

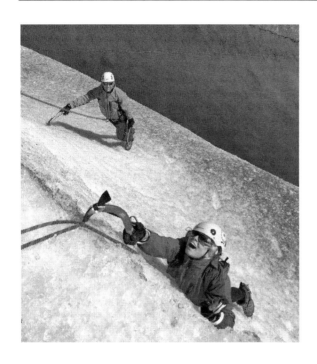

Dad + Daughter enjoying life minus 20 lbs., four years after weight loss with Z-Fast Maintenance keeping it under 185 lbs. to ice climb that mountain!

John says, "I had NO time to exercise and NO time for diets. I only had time NOT to EAT. FASTING WORKS." In Z-FAST, John shares the story of his successful fasting weight loss, the three personalized, proven methods for fasting, and the many health-boosting benefits that come with what has been discovered to be a natural way of eating. This book contains the answers for all those people who have asked over the years, *"Hey Johnny Z, can you write that fasting thing down for me?"*

As a busy medical device executive with a demanding career, John has discovered the secret to what it takes to balance a vibrant and full life. John has been happily married for over 26 years, has raised three daughters with his wife, and enjoys living in Southern California as an avid surfer. John is often described by those who know him best as unbelievably innovative, highly motivated, and a fun-spirited guy. Since he never takes "NO!" for an answer, the Z-FAST was born!

For more information, contact Johnny Z at jz@johnzehren.net and visit the website ZFAST.US.

We would love to hear about your success using the Z-FAST methods and add it to our growing list of successes stories highlighted at ZFAST.US! And don't forget to please leave a book review on Amazon. 😊

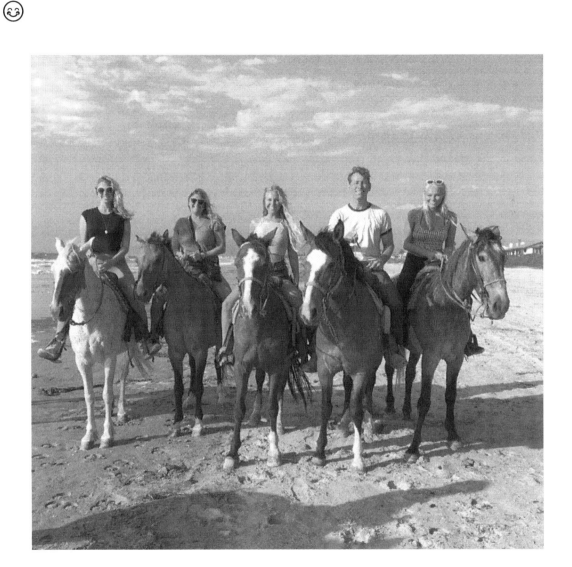

My family in Ensenada, Mexico right before the big gallop!

Losing and maintaining my weight has allowed happiness, health, respect, longevity all to be part of my new life as I want to be here for my wife and daughters for a long time.

RESOURCES

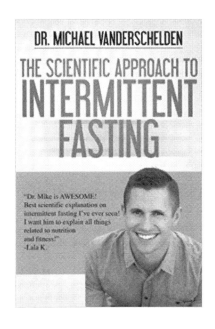

The Scientific Approach to Intermittent Fasting

Dr. Michael VanDerschelden, 2016

The best scientific description of fasting that I have read. He goes very deep into the science as only a medical doctor can. A great source for understanding the scientific approach, and he describes in great detail how to add intense exercise.

www.youtube.com/watch?v=5z9xkfILXsQ

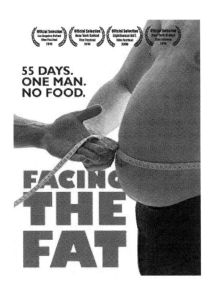

Facing the Fat

Directed by & starring Kenny Saylors, 2014

Amazon Prime film

"55 days without food: For years, Kenny Saylors was a fit, healthy man. Now, he's become an overweight, unhealthy shell of the man he once was. In an effort to turn his life around, Kenny accepts a challenge — 55 days on a strictly water-based no-food diet. *Facing the Fat* follows Kenny's journey to conquer obesity."

www.amazon.com/Facing-Fat-Kenny-Saylors/dp/B01MQR4ABI

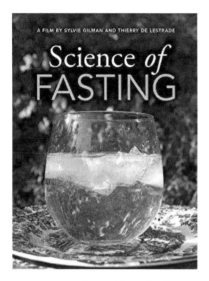

Science of Fasting

Studio Arte France, 2016

Directed by Sylvie Gilman & Thierry de Lestrade

Amazon Prime film

"Young biologists from the University of Southern California have overturned conventional wisdom and used molecular biology to demonstrate the powerful effects of fasting. This research suggests a wide-ranging potential, which could include treatments for the disease of the century, cancer. If these scientists are right, maybe our approach to disease and treatment will need a rethink."

www.amazon.com/Science-Fasting-Sylvie-Gilman/dp/B075848T5T

MORE RESOURCES

"10 Evidence-Based Health Benefits of Intermittent Fasting." *Healthline*, Healthline Media, www.healthline.com/nutrition/10-health-benefits-of-intermittent-fasting

"Are There Any Proven Benefits to Fasting?" Johns Hopkins Health Review, www.johnshopkinshealthreview.com/issues/spring-summer-2016/articles/are-there-any-proven-benefits-to-fasting

Bacon, Linda, and Aphramor, Lucy. "Weight Science: Evaluating the Evidence for a Paradigm Shift," *Nutrition Journal*, BioMed Central, 2011

"Can Coffee Increase Your Metabolism and Help You Burn Fat?" *Healthline*, Healthline Media, www.healthline.com/nutrition/coffee-increase-metabolism#section3

"Consider fasting for better health 10 Unbelievable Diet Rules Backed by Science." *The Fast Diet*, thefastdiet.co.uk/forums/topic/consider-fasting-for-better-health-10-unbelievable-diet-rules-backed-by-science/

"Energy Expenditure of Walking and Running," published in Medicine & Science in *Sports & Exercise*.

"Fasting and growth hormone." *Diet Doctor*, 15 Dec. 2017, www.dietdoctor.com/fasting-and-growth-hormone

"Fasting diet: Can it improve my heart health?" Mayo Clinic, Mayo Foundation for Medical Education and Research, 28 Sept. 2017, www.mayoclinic.org/diseases-conditions/heart-disease /expert-answers/fasting-diet/faq-20058334

"Fasting-like diet turns the immune system against cancer." *USC News*, 5 Feb. 2018, news.usc.edu/103972/fasting-like-diet-turns-the-immune-system-against-cancer/

Haridy, Rich. "Harvard Study Uncovers Why Fasting Can Lead to a Longer and Healthier Life." New Atlas – New Technology & Science News, *New Atlas*, 6 Nov. 2017, newatlas.com/fasting-increase-lifespan-mitochondria-harvard/52058/

Hartman, Veldhuis, Johnson, Lee, Alberti, Samojik, & Thorner (1992). "Augmented growth hormone (GH) secretory bursts frequency and amplitude mediate enhanced GH secretion during a two-day fast in normal man." *The Journal of Clinical Endocrinology and Metabolism*. 1992 Apr; 74(4); 757–765.
DOI 10.1210/jcem.74.4.1548337
www.ncbi.nlm.nih.gov/pubmed/1548337

"Heart Disease." Centers for Disease Control and Prevention, Centers for Disease Control and Prevention, 28 Nov. 2017, www.cdc.gov/heartdisease/facts.htm

Ho, Veldhuis, Johnson, Furlanetto, Evans, Alberti, & Thorner (1988). "Fasting enhances growth hormone secretion and amplifies the complex rhythms of growth hormone secretion in man." The Journal of Clinical Investigation. 1988 Apr; 81(4); 968–975. DOI: 10.1172/JCI113450.
www.ncbi.nlm.nih.gov/pmc/articles/PMC329619

"How Long Can a Person Survive without Food?" *Scientific American*, www.scientificamerican.com/article/how-long-can-a-person-sur/

"How Many Calories Are You Really Burning?" *Runner's World*, 4 Feb. 2016, www.runnersworld.com/weight-loss/how-many-calories-are-you-really-burning

http://eip.uindy.edu/crossings/publications/Interfaith%20Conversations-1.pdf

"Hungry stomach hormone promotes growth of new brain cells." *New Scientist*, www.newscientist.com/article/2128695-hungry-stomach-hormone-promotes-growth-of-new-brain-cells/

"Intermittent Fasting: 3 Little-Known Changes You Can Trigger." The Health Sciences Academy, 29 Mar. 2016, thehealthsciencesacademy.org/health-tips/intermittent-fasting/

Mattson, M P, et al. "Meal size and frequency affect neuronal plasticity and vulnerability to disease: cellular and molecular mechanisms." *Journal of Neurochemistry*, U.S. National Library of Medicine, Feb. 2003, www.ncbi.nlm.nih.gov/pubmed/12558961

Mike Wilson Fasting and Exercise Program. Sign up for a WEBINAR. http://capemayfitness.com/intermittentfasting&training.php

Peart, Karen N. "Anti-Inflammatory mechanism of dieting and fasting revealed." *YaleNews*, 19 Dec. 2017, news.yale.edu/2015/02/16/anti-inflammatory-mechanism-dieting-and-fasting-revealed

"Prevalence of Obesity Among Adults and Youth: United States, 2011–2014." Centers for Disease Control and Prevention, Centers for Disease Control and Prevention, 28 Oct. 2015, www.cdc.gov/nchs/data/databriefs/db219.html

"Resting energy expenditure in short-term starvation is increased as a result of an increase in serum norepinephrine." Am J Clin Nutr.; 71(6):1511-5. Zauner C, Schneeweiss B.

Stipp, D. (2013, January 01). "How Intermittent Fasting Might Help You Live a Longer and Healthier Life." Retrieved from https://www.scientificamerican.com/article/how-intermittent-fasting-might-help-you-live-longer-healthier-life/

Team, Heart and Vascular. "Fasting: How Does It Affect Your Heart and Blood Pressure?" Health Essentials from Cleveland Clinic, Health Essentials from Cleveland Clinic, 20 July 2017, health.clevelandclinic.org/fasting-how-does-it-affect-your-heart-and-blood-pressure/

"The best ways to cut calories from your diet." Mayo Clinic, Mayo Foundation for Medical Education and Research, 11 Apr. 2015, www.mayoclinic.org/healthy-lifestyle/weight-loss/in-depth/calories/art-20048065

"Why Jews Fast." TheTorah.com, thetorah.com/why-jews-fast/

Wolpert, Stuart. "Dieting Does Not Work, UCLA Researchers Report." *UCLA Newsroom*, 3 Apr. 2007, newsroom.ucla.edu/releases/Dieting-Does-Not-Work-UCLA-Researchers-7832

Youm, Yun-Hee, et al. "The ketone metabolite β-Hydroxybutyrate blocks NLRP3 inflammasome–mediated inflammatory disease." *Nature News*, Nature Publishing Group, 16 Feb. 2015, www.nature.com/articles/nm.3804

Printed in Great Britain
by Amazon